MATERNITY ABROAD

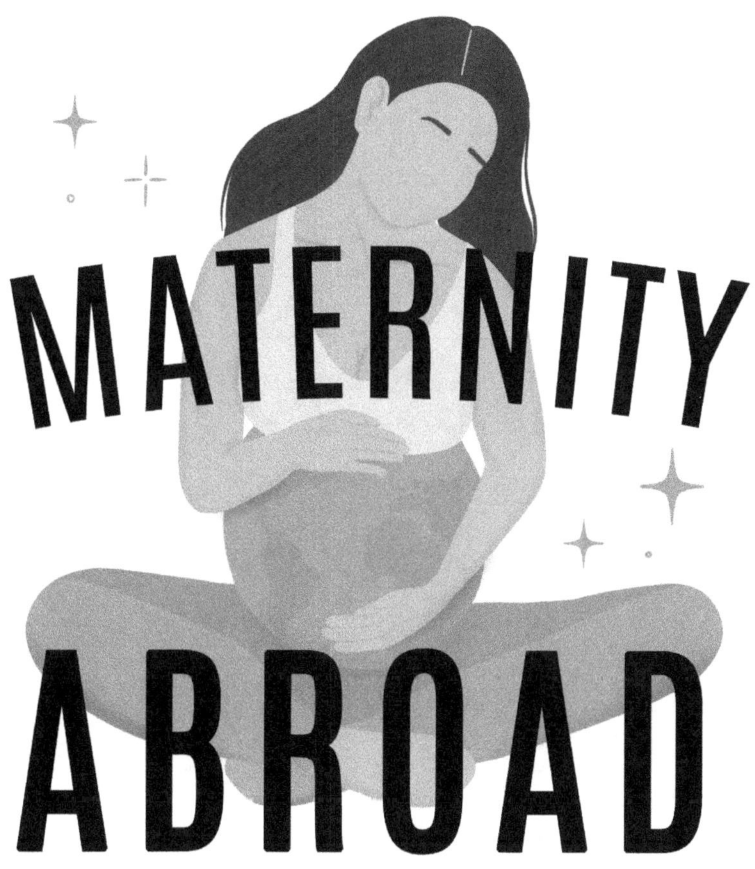

MATERNITY ABROAD

BECOMING A MOTHER IN A FOREIGN LAND

JESSICA GABRIELZYK

PUBLISHED BY KEEP IT SIMPLE PUBLISHING

Maternity Abroad

Becoming a Mother in a Foreign Land

Copyright © 2024 by Jessica Gabrielzyk

Published by Keep It Simple Publishing

ISBN: 978-2-9701848-0-5

ACKNOWLEDGEMENTS

First and foremost, I would like to thank my family for their unwavering support and love throughout this journey.

I am deeply grateful to all the mothers who allowed their stories to be told in this book and generously shared their real names. Your bravery and openness have enriched this work immensely.

Additionally, I would like to express my heartfelt gratitude to the international specialists who provided their professional advice for the special section at the end of the book. Your insights and expertise have been invaluable in enriching this work and offering practical guidance to readers facing similar experiences. Thank you for your contributions and support.

Lastly, I extend a heartfelt thank you to my obstetrician, Dr. Ana Sofia Fernandes, and my midwife, Cláudia Boticas, from Porto, Portugal, who made my pregnancy an incredible experience. Despite our cultural differences, you warmly welcomed and cared for me exceptionally well. Without your dedication and support, I probably wouldn't have written this book. Your exemplary work as healthcare professionals provided me with the confidence and strength I needed during this important time. Thank you for being such wonderful caregivers and making this chapter of my life so memorable.

CONTENTS

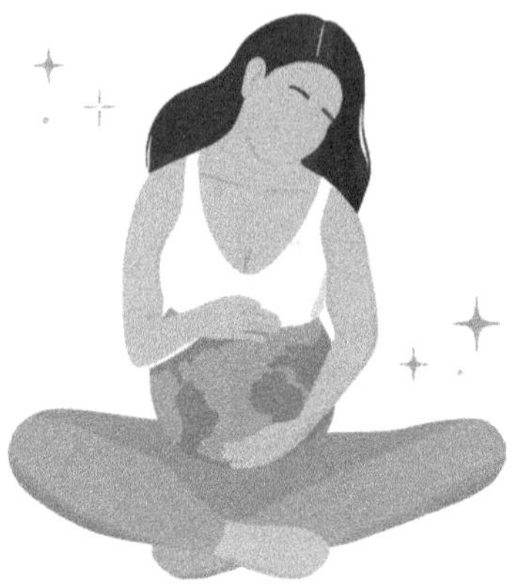

INTRODUCTION

Do you remember the first time you held a baby? I sure do. My eyes were as wide as saucers as I held my friend's newborn like a ticking bomb. Babies are fragile, innocent Rubik's cubes—you need to solve them while they're doing the same thing because they don't know themselves either. And, well ... they're noisy too. Especially when they're hungry, sleepy, tired, cold, too warm, overstimulated, bored, have an itchy toe, or anything, really.

As you can probably guess, I was never a 'let me hold your baby' kind of person. I was the one who would gift parents a giant, plush unicorn (true story)—you know, the kind of gift that's more of a hassle than a help, as any *Friends* fan would know.

Yet, when the idea of starting a family began to feel like a natural step in my ten-year relationship with my husband, things changed. We've always been that couple who loves a juicy adventure. From traveling the charming streets of Copenhagen and vibrant cityscapes of Melbourne to soaking in the bustling energy of Osaka and New York City's iconic vibe, we've done it all. And if no one stops me, I could keep going about the amazing places we've visited. We just didn't stop.

However, as we set out on this new and beautiful path, I began to realize how different this journey was going to be abroad. The thing is, back in Brazil, when someone decided to have a baby, family and friends were the go-to for everything baby-related. Need advice? Neighbor Maria is on speed dial. Looking for hand-me-downs? Cousin João's garage is a treasure trove.

That was my epiphany—I was utterly unprepared to have a baby. In general, life in Portugal was quite different from my Brazilian home. When pregnancy and parenting are thrown into the mix, things become even more complex. Most of us expatriates learn this the hard way, often only having our partners to lean on for support. And if you're a single mother, that's another layer of terrifying.

Motherhood was more daunting than accepting that *pão de queijo* (delicious Brazilian cheese breads) aren't readily available everywhere. Just like me, mothers from all over the world face similar dilemmas. Regardless of our backgrounds, being pregnant in a foreign country is a unique and often challenging experience.

When I moved to Portugal in April 2023, life was full of surprises. Just weeks before receiving my positive pregnancy test, I was leisurely sipping *ginja*, a cherished Portuguese cherry liqueur, in a quaint alley of Porto. My biggest worry was making it to Jardim do Morro in time to watch the sunset. Not long after, I was plunged into the existential crises of motherhood.

Outsiders may think that adjusting to a cultural shift from Brazil to Portugal should be easy. In fact, even the language differences between Brazil and Portugal might seem trivial to an untrained ear. It's all

Portuguese, right? It can't be that hard to adjust. However, the variations are as distinct as Americans saying "afternoon" and Australians casually using "arvo" for the same time of day. While a lot of words and phrases sounded similar, I found myself constantly decoding a whole new set of cultural cues, each day presenting its own unique linguistic challenges.

Honestly, verbal faux pas just became a part of my daily routine here: Wake up, go to work, say something wrong that will make me cringe for years to come (like the time I was attempting to speak French and said *moiselle* instead of *mademoiselle*. Yes, I know *moiselle* isn't even a word! Oh, that haunts me). Or, the many times I pretended to understand what someone was saying because I was too shy to ask them to repeat it. I would just reply "yes" because it seemed fitting. When I look back, I have no idea if the question was something that required a "yes or no" answer or something like, "How old are you?"

But nothing tops the mix-up I had with my obstetrician. So, I called this packet of powder that looked like sugar a *sachê*. Turns out, over here they call it a *saqueta*. We went back and forth for thirty minutes before we figured out that we were talking about the same thing! We eventually laughed it off, but let's be real: Mixing up meds when you're pregnant is no joke. It wasn't just about me anymore.

And the shift from just trotting around the globe to dealing with the physical changes of pregnancy was something else! Let me tell you this— they shouldn't even call it "sleep" when you're pregnant. If you've been there, you know exactly what I'm talking about. And if you're planning for your first baby, well, prepare to kiss a good night's sleep goodbye.

When you're pregnant, you don't really sleep deeply; you're almost always half awake, ready to jump up at the slightest sound. Part of it is the constant worry and anticipation, but there's also the physical discomfort.

Trying to find a comfortable position with a growing belly and constant backaches is a challenge in itself, and then there's the need to get up for frequent bathroom trips. It's a perfect recipe for sleepless nights ... and vivid dreams (that's a thing we go through too! I still remember a couple of mine).

Those sleepless nights hit me way harder than I thought they would. And here I was, thinking that keeping a cactus alive was tough—ha! Try stepping into motherhood in a foreign country. It's like executing a high dive and realizing halfway down that you forgot to check if there's water in the pool.

Entering this new landscape as an expectant mother was an adventure tinged with anxiety. One day, I was learning how to order decaf coffee in a local *padaria* (bakery) without receiving judgmental looks (in Portugal, decaffeinated coffee is virtually synonymous with plain hot water). The next, I was decoding baby essentials in a language that, though familiar now, at the time still seemed to play by its own rules. This constant adjustment reminded me of my days traveling, where every new place brought with it a blend of excitement and challenges, but with the added responsibility of taking care of a fragile newborn.

It's not that this whole life abroad thing was new to me. As I explained before, I've been around—from Australia's sun-kissed beaches to Ireland's lush greenery. I had danced through life's curveballs quite often. But even this nomadic resilience paled in comparison to the seismic shift of becoming a parent. Moving abroad is a challenge on its own. There's the language barrier, the culture adjustment, the paperwork, and then there's the emotional side of it, brought about by the move away from home and family. Navigating a pregnancy in this context is a whole other story.

Being away from your familiar support network during such a vulnerable time transforms what is typically a shared joy into a more solitary journey.

It wasn't just a new chapter; it was an entirely different book. No matter how many tales I'd heard, or how much advice I'd gathered, knowing I would have to care for someone so vulnerable was like stepping onto a thrilling, terrifying stage without a script. Mispronounce a street name in Dublin? That's laughable. Misinterpret a baby's cry? That's panic mode.

When in Rome—or Portugal, in this case—I might have tried to 'do as the Romans do.' But Romans likely didn't rely on Google to desperately try not to botch changing diapers. The prenatal course nurse tried to reassure me with, "Your baby can sense your anxiety," which honestly didn't help. I felt like I was poised to raise the human version of a jittery Chihuahua.

Experiencing motherhood in a new country taught me that while being multilingual is great for parties, it complicates parsing through baby advice. From ancient remedies like rubbing garlic on the baby's feet to bathing them strictly at noon, I felt more equipped for a stint in vampire defense than parenting.

And then so many tasks were waiting to welcome me, like juggling insurance covers, visa issues, and hospital protocols on top of all the typical pregnancy challenges.

As someone who has navigated the challenges of maternity abroad, I say with all sincerity: You've got this. Seriously! Your decision to embark on this journey while living far away from your comfort zone certainly deserves applause. I've exchanged stories with other expatriate mothers, and each narrative reinforced the incredible resilience of these women— now you're one of them.

Do you know how I know? Because you're holding the guidebook for just that: *Maternity Abroad: Becoming a Mother in a Foreign Land.* Whether you're planning your move, already unpacking in a new country, or simply curious about what it's like to become a mom on foreign soil, this book is for you.

I've packed these pages with everything you need to know, shared by those who have walked this path before you. You'll find stories from moms who have experienced the highs and lows of motherhood away from their home country, plus heaps of advice and resources to help you along the way.

Here's a sneak peek of what's inside:

• **Welcome to The World, Little One:** How do you deal with the local healthcare system? What is the best way to provide prenatal care when you're miles from home? We'll help you figure all that out and prepare you mentally, physically, and logistically for your new arrival.

• **Establishing a Strong Foundation: Health Insurance, Legalities, and a Support Network**: Dealing with different health insurance rules, birthright citizenship regulations, dual nationality questions, parental leave rights, legal paperwork, and building a strong support network can be a major headache, but I've got you covered.

• **The Birthing Experience Abroad:** Ever wonder how birthing practices differ around the world? I've got the inside scoop on hospitals, birthing centers, and even home births in various countries, plus tips on advocating for your birthing plan, wherever you are.

• **Postpartum Support and Practices:** Those first few weeks with your baby are precious. We'll guide you through finding support and adapting to postpartum practices in your new community, so you can focus on recovery and bonding.

• **Pediatric Healthcare and Childcare:** Pediatrician or general practitioner? Who's going to look after your baby when you're at work or need those extra hours for yourself?

• **Resources and Support:** Finally, we'll conclude with a Q&A with international specialists to help you understand the journey you've undertaken.

So, without further ado, welcome to our slice of maternity abroad—a haven of real-life stories to comfort, guide, and entertain. If you've ever doubted yourself or used 'baby brain' as an excuse for forgetting your keys, remember, it's real and you're not alone. So, grab a cup of your favorite coffee (or tea, but I'm sticking to coffee because with a toddler at home, I need it!), settle in, and let's start this adventure together.

Here's to embracing the beautiful chaos of raising global citizens—one story, one lesson, and one joy at a time!

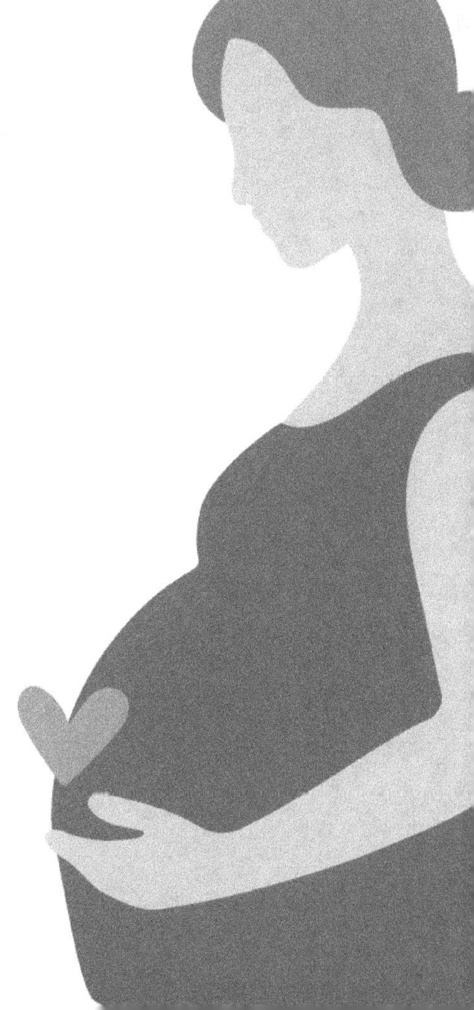

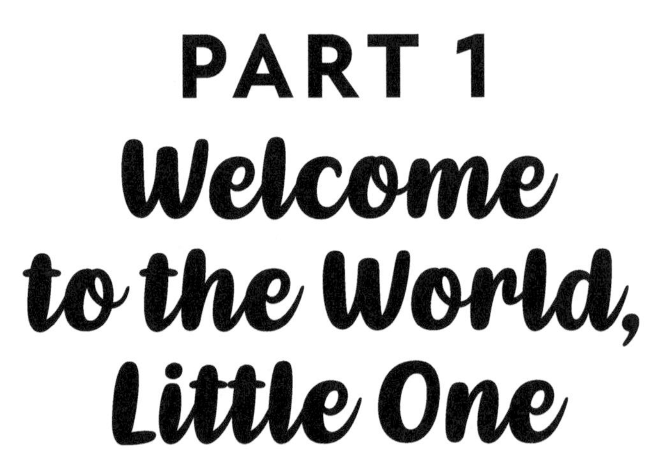

PART 1
Welcome to the World, Little One

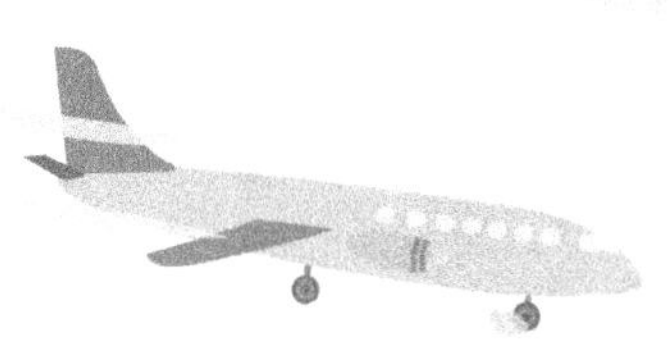

Join me as we go through the incredible experience of becoming a mother far from home. In this chapter, we'll explore the intricacies of managing foreign **healthcare systems and unravel prenatal care.** This isn't just a guide—it's a helping hand from friends who have trodden this path. Because let's face it: Giving birth in a new country is a path we're all stumbling through together. It's not going to be easy, but this guide aims to make things a little less chaotic for you, so you can welcome your little bundle of joy without being constantly on edge.

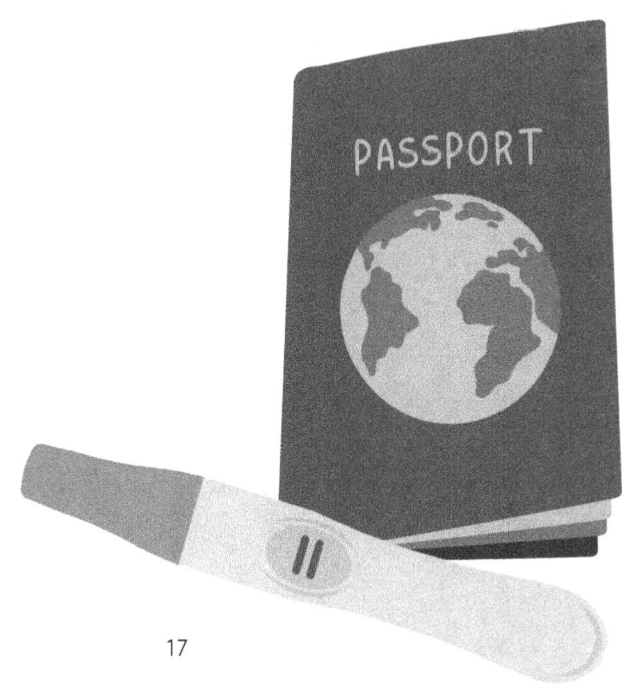

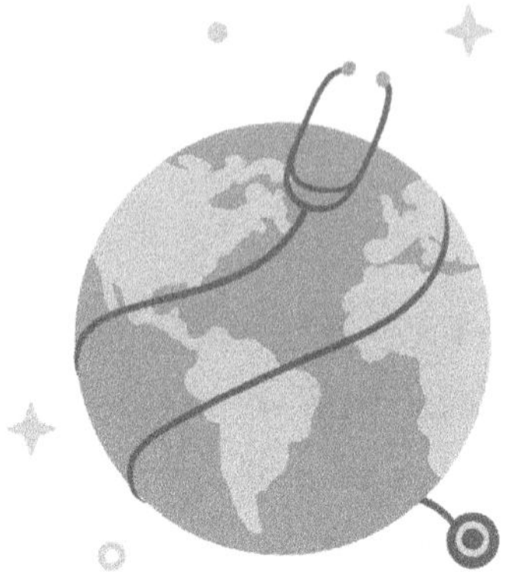

UNDERSTANDING HEALTHCARE WHEN YOU'RE FAR FROM HOME

Imagine we're sitting down with our coffees, and you're about to move abroad. You ask, "How does healthcare work over there?" Well, it's a bit like trying to find the best coffee in a new city. Every place does it a bit differently, and finding your favorite spot can take some trial and error.

WHAT'S THE DEAL WITH HEALTHCARE AROUND THE WORLD?

First off, you've got places like the UK, which use the **Beveridge model.**[1] In other words, the government in these countries handles healthcare, kind of like they oversee public libraries and roads. Everything is funded through taxes. Larissa, an immigrant mother living in London, who gave birth to her son through the public healthcare system (a.k.a., NHS or National Healthcare System), had a funny take on it: "Everyone uses the NHS. Well, except maybe the royals and the Beckhams. It works."

Still, getting used to your new reality may be easier said than done. Luana Messias, a mother of two, has been using the public healthcare system in Australia since 2011. She shares, "If you're an international mother who isn't very familiar with the public system here, it's about trusting it, right? As Brazilians, we tend to distrust the public system for numerous reasons back home. But here, it works very well."

Not everyone finds this to be an easy adjustment, though. Think about it—only approximately 53% of Brazilians really trust their healthcare system. So, imagine the leap it takes to trust a system in an entirely new country, where it is natural to approach everything with some caution. This challenge isn't unique to Brazil; it happens all over the world. For instance, 36% of Russians trust their healthcare system, while the numbers are 55% in Nigeria, 47% in Argentina, and 50% in Colombia.[2]

Then you've got the **Bismarck model**, which is more like a dinner club where everyone chips in for the meal. Countries like Germany, Japan, and France use this system, where everyone pays into insurance funds that cover healthcare costs.[1] Japan requires "mandatory coverage for anyone who permanently resides in the country for three months or more. This includes both Japanese and non-Japanese citizens."[3]

Flavia Imamura, who moved to Okinawa a little less than a decade ago, explains, "Health here is not public; it is not 100% free. We always pay. In fact, we pay 30%, and the government pays 70%, which would be our health plan. Residents are obliged to enter this plan, which is already deducted from salary payment."

The **National Health Insurance Model**, which is a mix of the Beveridge and Bismarck models, is used in places like Canada. Think of it as choosing between a flat white or an espresso at different cafes. In this system, the government funds healthcare, but private companies provide the services.

It's a hybrid model that combines public funding with private delivery, and it works smoothly for the most part.[1] An immigrant mother of two, Carina believes that the Canadian healthcare system works. "Here, you need to see your family doctor for everything. Back in Brazil, if I needed to see a specialist, I had private health insurance through my work, and I could just go ahead and book it. Here, it's different. Your family doctor handles everything, from gynecological exams to looking after your kids. However, in two instances, navigating this system was a struggle. My daughter had gastrointestinal issues, and getting a referral for her to see a specialist was a thorough back-and-forth game of persistence. The same thing happened to me when I started experiencing menopause symptoms and wanted a gynecologist to look after me. On the positive side, once you have a referral, you have access to your specialist for life."

Finally, we have the unfortunate **Uninsured Model**, which is straightforward but tough. In this system, if you can afford to pay for healthcare, you're good; if not, it's a real challenge. It's like having to buy a pricey coffee without any guarantee it'll taste good. Countries with this model have no widespread health coverage or insurance system, so individuals must cover their medical expenses out-of-pocket, which can be a significant burden for those without sufficient financial resources.[1] Alessandra Ravasi shared her thoughts on the healthcare system: "In the US, having paid health insurance is the way to go. It's the best option. I have nothing but gratitude for the doctors I've seen in Virginia. As for the hospitals, I can't complain either. I've always used my husband's paid health insurance. Even with my Multiple Sclerosis (MS), if I were in Brazil, I wouldn't have access to the advanced treatments and medication that I have in the US."

TIPS FOR HANDLING HEALTHCARE ABROAD

Now, say you're about to embark on this big adventure of planning a family abroad. Here's how to make sure you find good coffee … er … I mean, good healthcare:

• **Do Your Homework:** Take some time to learn about the healthcare system in your new country. How does insurance work over here? What's covered? What's not? Doing this can save you a lot of surprises. Start with some online research on government healthcare websites. Join forums for transplants like yourself to hear what others have to say; visit local clinics to pick up pamphlets; ask questions; and check out local clinics' reviews for additional insights. Many of these places offer translators to help with language barriers, and in some cases, pamphlets are available in other languages too.

• **Get Registered:** Find a local doctor or a health clinic as soon as you get there, especially if you need a referral for anything.

• **Be Prepared for Anything:** Memorize the emergency numbers and the quickest route to the nearest medical facility.

• **When in Rome:** Embrace the local healthcare customs. Talk to local doctors or visit a healthcare clinic to get the best advice. Again, joining groups and online forums dedicated to expatriates can also provide helpful insights. Check out official health department websites and local embassies for detailed guides and resources.

• **Watch Your Budget:** Understand what you'll have to pay out of your own pocket to avoid unexpected expenses. Handling healthcare in a new country is about keeping an open mind, asking lots of questions, and maybe even embracing some local flavors—whether that's healthcare or coffee. So, let's sip on that and get you ready for your big move!

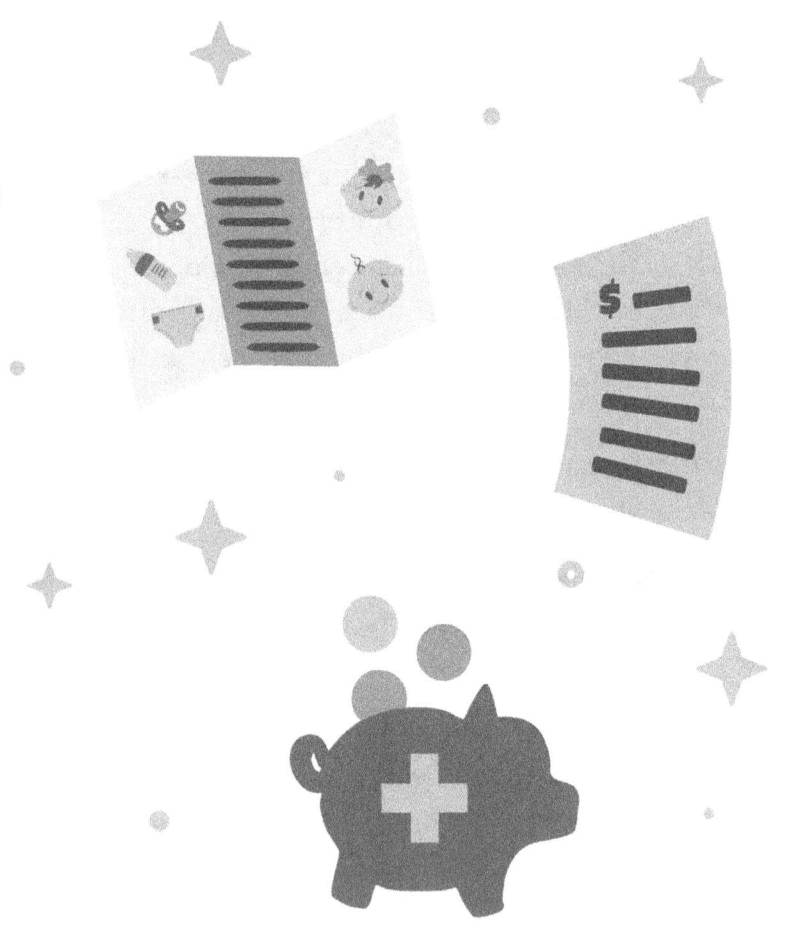

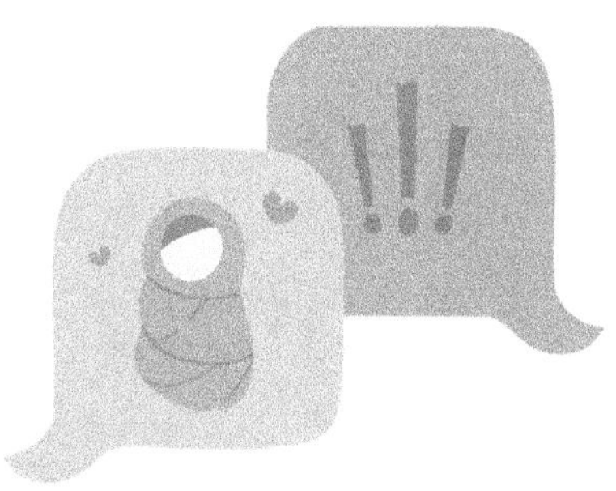

Finding Humanized Care in the Land of Port Wine: A real-life tale

Sitting in a crowded emergency room, feeling the familiar sharp pain from a recurrent urinary infection while also being pregnant, Cintia blinked, baffled at the nurse standing in front of her. *It couldn't be real, could it?*

She gulped, trying to find the words to ask, "A cup of tea?"

The nurse smiled at her. "You look like you need a cup of tea."

Urinary infections had been far more frequent during the course of her pregnancy than they had for any of her family members. No wonder she felt like the infection had clouded her judgment, making her trust her doctor's recommendation to give this new hospital a shot. *A nurse kindly offering a cup of tea? This simply could not be real.*

You see, Centro Materno Infantil do Norte in Porto, also known as CMIN, wasn't the closest hospital to her house. But the closest one had already let her down, so she figured this new hospital was worth checking out. A single experience with a doctor at the first hospital had left her emotionally scarred. "I was very poorly attended to by a doctor who was giving a class to a resident next door. She put the speculum on me to do the evaluation. When I complained that it hurt, she turned to me and said, 'Now it hurts, right?' She was really rude. She's a terrible doctor," Cintia recalled.

Cintia came from a private healthcare setting in her home country, and despite consultation delays in crowded medical offices, she had never experienced such a lack of empathy. Although her experience with the public system in Portugal was disappointing, she didn't dismiss the entire system, as she had also encountered compassionate and attentive doctors. Her issue wasn't with the public system itself; it was with the specific doctor who had treated her poorly.

She had lived for a short period in Portugal when she was only 17, so it's not like everything was brand new to her. She decided to return to her home country only to come back years later. At this stage of her life, putting her pregnancy in safe hands meant everything.

It wasn't her first pregnancy, but it would be her first baby. After marrying the love of her life in Brazil, she had a heartbreaking miscarriage. "The baby stopped developing at nine weeks, and the little heart stopped at twelve," Cintia shared, her voice heavy with sorrow.

When she returned to Portugal years later, her desire to be a mother rekindled. After another miscarriage in 2022 and learning that her small ovaries were making conception difficult, Cintia began to experience depression and panic attacks. But a trip to Madeira Island changed everything. "I wasn't trying to get pregnant, but I didn't prevent it either, and on Madeira Island, I felt an unusual ovulation pain," she recounted, hinting at fate's hand with a rainbow keychain she purchased there. Soon, she was pregnant with Arthur, the boy with caramel blond hair who was destined to charm the world (spoiler alert!)

However, Cintia's pregnancy was fraught with challenges, including repeated urinary infections. Recovering from her bad experience with her first doctor, she sought advice from Dr. Graça, whom she affectionately called Dr. Giselle Bündchen because she had the exact surname as the Brazilian model. Dr. Graça told her to try CMIN, and Cintia, being the strong soul that she is, didn't give up on the public system.

Cintia felt a mix of fear and hope as she navigated the unfamiliar public healthcare system in Portugal. Each visit to the hospital was a reminder of her past loss, but also a step toward her dream of motherhood. The anxiety of another potential disappointment weighed heavily on her, but she persevered.

She accepted the cup of tea while waiting to be examined. In the ultrasound room, the same caring nurse was there to confirm another urinary infection. Despite the setback, the nurse's kindness provided some comfort. At the end of the examination, the nurse printed the ultrasound picture of her baby for her to take home.

Holding the picture, Cintia felt a renewed sense of determination. Each small victory, like the printed image, was a reminder that she was closer to her goal. The journey was tough, but her resolve to bring her baby into the world kept her moving forward.

"I was in love with the place by the time I left," she admitted. Not only did she stick with this trusted hospital until childbirth, but she also narrates her wonderful experiences with a wide smile and a giggle here and there.

Cintia's journey shows that finding the right support system in healthcare settings is a key part of navigating pregnancy abroad. And hey, if your current doctor or hospital isn't cutting it, don't stress! You can always shop around for better ones. Remember, you're not stuck with any one doctor or hospital. Think of it like dating, but with way less awkward small talk and no bad coffee meetups. Your peace of mind is worth the search!

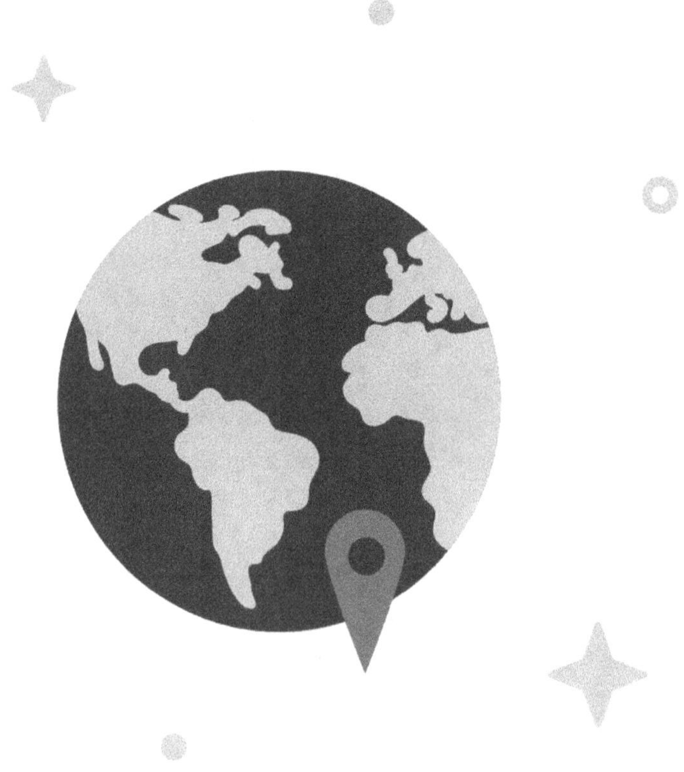

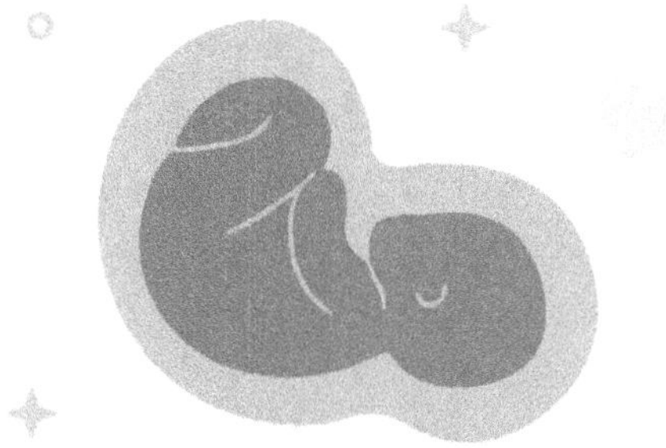

UNDERSTANDING PRENATAL CARE

I have to be honest here: While I had some idea of what to expect during my pregnancy, like regular doctor visits, a couple of blood tests, and definitely some ultrasounds, I was totally clueless about many other things like the need for glucose tests and identifying chromosomal problems. Discovering prenatal care was like uncovering and stepping into a whole new world of surprises.

Prenatal care, in simple terms, includes the checkups and tests you are required to undergo throughout your pregnancy. It's crucial because it helps keep both you and your baby healthy by enabling your healthcare provider to catch any potential health problems proactively. Early treatment can solve many issues and prevent new ones from developing. However, availability and requirements for prenatal care can vary from country to country, so it's important to understand what your specific location offers and recommends.

Your doctor or midwife will set up a schedule for your prenatal visits. If you're over 35, or if your pregnancy is considered high-risk due to conditions like diabetes or high blood pressure, they'll likely want to see you more often. And as your due date approaches, you can expect these visits to become even more frequent, since they are necessary to make sure everything is on track.[4] Keep in mind that the frequency and scheduling of these visits might vary depending on the country's healthcare system.

How does the type of healthcare system affect my prenatal care service access?

That's the big question, isn't it? The truth is *your access to prenatal services will vary.* In some places, you might need a referral from a general practitioner to see an obstetrician, while in others you can directly visit a specialist. Understanding these pathways will save you time and stress.

• **Referrals and Appointments:** In some healthcare systems, you'll need a primary care doctor's referral to see a specialist like an OB-GYN, which means your first step is finding a reliable general practitioner. Sorting this out early helps prevent delays in your prenatal care.

• **Specialist Access:** In countries with more flexible systems, you might be able to book appointments directly with prenatal specialists. This can be a quicker route, but it might come with higher out-of-pocket costs if you're using private insurance.

Managing Prenatal Health and Well-Being

Part of me wants to tell you to go ahead and indulge in all those yummy treats you're craving for the next nine months—chocolate, cheese, pizza ... maybe even a bucket of iced vanilla coffee with whipped cream on top (yes, that's my go-to summer treat). But we both know that's not good advice. A balanced diet is crucial not just for the baby, but for you too. I get it—when you move to another country, you just want to indulge in all the delicious local offerings. And the cravings ... oh, those *pastéis de nata*! If you haven't tried a Portuguese *pastel de nata*, beware—it's the ultimate temptation. A crispy, flaky pastry cup filled with creamy vanilla custard, this yummy dessert is topped with a sprinkle of cinnamon. It's so mouth-watering that walking past the bakery near my house feels like a punishment. I practically need horse blinders to avoid buying their entire stock daily!

But sweets aren't everything. There's the savory side too. Maybe you're a South American like me, and you've moved to a place where burgers and fries are as common as your everyday rice and beans. Or perhaps you're from the Netherlands, where the variety of breads and sandwiches is practically an art form (by the way, if you're from there, I'm a huge fan of your culinary scene!). Now, you've moved to a place where hearty soups with noodles, steamed vegetables, and boiled eggs are the norm. Suddenly, you're faced with a whole new set of dietary guidelines, and it feels like trying to decipher a foreign menu where the only thing you recognize is water. No need to panic, though; let's tackle this together!

Adjusting your nutrition and diet while embracing your new culinary surroundings can be both challenging and exciting. Here's how to make it work:

LOCAL DIETARY RECOMMENDATIONS FOR PREGNANT WOMEN

1. **Understanding Local Guidelines:** First, get to know the local dietary rules. Different countries have their own set of beliefs about what's best for expectant moms, often based on local foods and customs. For example, in Japan, some types of sushi are completely acceptable during pregnancy, while in the US, they might treat you like you just suggested skydiving with your unborn child if you want to gorge on this popular seafood dish.

2. **Nutrient-Rich Foods:** Look out for local foods rich in essential nutrients like folic acid, iron, calcium, and DHA. These are your pregnancy superfoods. Many countries have their own nutritional powerhouses, like calcium-rich dairy in Europe or omega-3-loaded fish in coastal areas.

3. **Consult An Expert:** Don't be shy about asking for help. Local nutritionists and healthcare providers can offer tailored advice that aligns with your new environment while keeping your pregnant body healthy. They're like personal general practitioners dedicated to your diet and helping you find the best available nutrients.

FINDING FAMILIAR FOODS AND ADAPTING TO LOCAL CUISINE

1. **Locating Familiar Foods:** Craving that crunchy peanut butter from home? Most big cities have international grocery stores where you can find familiar brands. If not, there's always the magic of online shopping. Make use of the internet, which allows peanut butter and other goodies to arrive at your doorstep like a culinary care package from your past life. But what if you can't find what you're craving? In that case, you could

try making it yourself. If you're anything like me, an amazing chef with my own fancy French title—a *délusionnel chef* (a name my friends gave me after I nailed my attempt at making Brazilian styled *sfiha*, which they claimed was so good they insisted on celebrating with McDonald's)—you could try replicating recipes at home. Or, you might want to look for local alternatives with a similar nutrient and flavor profile.

2. **Exploring Local Markets:** Take a stroll through local markets as a great way to discover fresh produce and local delicacies. Plus, it can turn into a fun quest for picking ingredients that you can transform into delicious, nutrient-packed meals.

3. **Adapting Recipes:** Try putting a local twist on your favorite recipes. This can be a fun way to mix the familiar with the exotic. Can't find kale? Maybe there's a local leafy green that does the trick just as well.

With these tips, you'll be able to maintain a healthy diet while enjoying your new home's unique flavors. Happy eating!

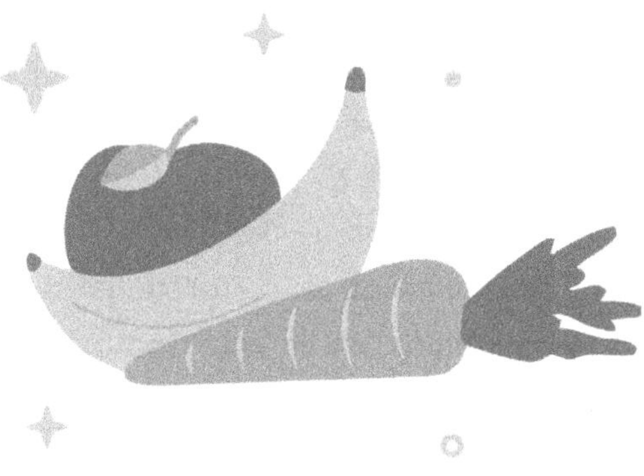

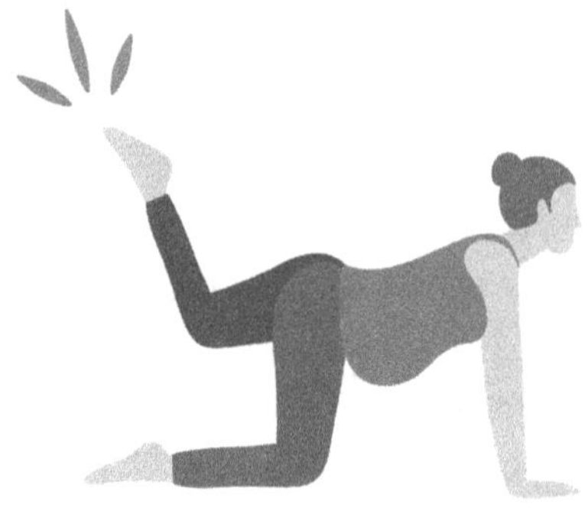

Exercise and Physical Activity

I wish I could share a secret recipe for endless energy during pregnancy, but honestly, I don't have one. I was that pregnant person who seemed to have an energy drink on drip. I had so much energy! (Don't worry; that's all in the past. Now, I'm mostly exhausted from chasing my toddler around, making sure she doesn't set the house on fire or decide the dog is her new chew toy.)

The reality is that every pregnancy is unique, just as each individual body behaves differently. Some people have boundless energy, while others feel tired all the time. It's perfectly normal. If you find yourself feeling more fatigued than usual, or if you experience symptoms like weakness, pale skin, rapid heartbeat, shortness of breath, or trouble concentrating, it's a good idea to talk to your doctor. These can sometimes be signs of anemia, which is common during pregnancy. So, listen to your body and don't hesitate to ask for medical advice to ensure you and your baby stay healthy and happy.[5]

Finding the perfect balance between rest and activity is the key to staying active during pregnancy. Both of these elements are refreshing and necessary! Whether you're in your home country or adjusting to a new one, maintaining a healthy exercise routine is just as crucial for you and your baby as your diet. Let's dive into how you can keep moving and grooving, no matter where you are.

FINDING THE RIGHT ACTIVITIES

1. **Local Classes and Groups:** One of the best ways to stay active is by joining local prenatal exercise classes. These offerings can range from prenatal yoga and Pilates to swimming and walking groups. Not only do these classes help you stay fit, but they're also fantastic for meeting other expectant mothers in your new community. It's a wonderful opportunity to make friends and bond with people who are on a similar journey and hence are equipped to support you emotionally. Plus, there's nothing like bonding over the shared struggles of swollen feet and midnight cravings!

2. **Exploring the Outdoors:** If you're living somewhere with beautiful parks or scenic walking paths, take advantage of them! A brisk walk in the fresh air can do wonders for your mood and health. And if you're lucky enough to be near a beach or mountains, gentle hikes can be both relaxing and invigorating. Just remember to keep the intensity at a comfortable level for you—no need to summit Everest right now!

ADAPTING TO THE CLIMATE

1. **Weather Considerations:** Moving to a new country often means adjusting to a different climate. If you're in a hot and humid place, early morning or late evening workouts might be best in order to avoid the midday heat. On the flip side, if you've moved to a cold region, layer up and keep your walks shorter to avoid the chill. And always listen to your body—it's your best guide.

2. **Indoor Options:** Sometimes, the weather just won't cooperate, or you might not feel safe venturing out. In these cases, indoor activities can be a lifesaver. Many countries offer prenatal workout videos online, and you can follow along from the comfort of your home. Whether it's yoga, light aerobics, or simple stretching exercises, staying active indoors is entirely possible and effective.

SAFETY FIRST

1. **Consulting Healthcare Providers:** Always check with your healthcare provider before starting any new exercise routine. This consideration is especially important if you're in a new country with different medical practices. A good healthcare provider can offer guidance that is tailored to your health needs and pregnancy stage, ensuring you and your baby stay safe and sound.

2. **Listening to Your Body:** Pregnancy isn't the time for extreme sports or pushing your limits. The goal is to stay active and healthy, not to set new personal records. Pay attention to how you feel during and after exercise. If something feels off, slow down or stop and consult your healthcare provider.

MAKING EXERCISE FUN

1. **Buddy System:** Exercising with a friend can help you stay disciplined. If you know other expectant moms, suggest meeting up for walks or classes. A dedicated workout buddy can keep you motivated and make the experience more enjoyable. Plus, it's a great way to swap tips and stories about pregnancy in your new home!

2. **Mixing It Up:** Don't be afraid to try new things. If your new country offers unique activities—like tai chi in a park in China or belly dancing in the Middle East—give them a shot! Staying active should be fun, and trying new exercises can be a delightful way to immerse yourself in the local culture.

Staying active during pregnancy doesn't have to be daunting, even when you're settling down in a new country. Embrace the opportunities your new environment offers, and remember, it's all about keeping it light and enjoyable. Every little bit helps, so keep moving, stay healthy, and enjoy the journey!

And let's not forget about the 'feel-good' hormones! Exercising releases endorphins, dopamine, and serotonin—those magical chemicals that boost your mood. This influx of happy hormones is a godsend when you're navigating the challenges of being alone in a new country. So, staying active isn't only good for your body; it also keeps your spirits high, making it easier to adapt to your new surroundings.

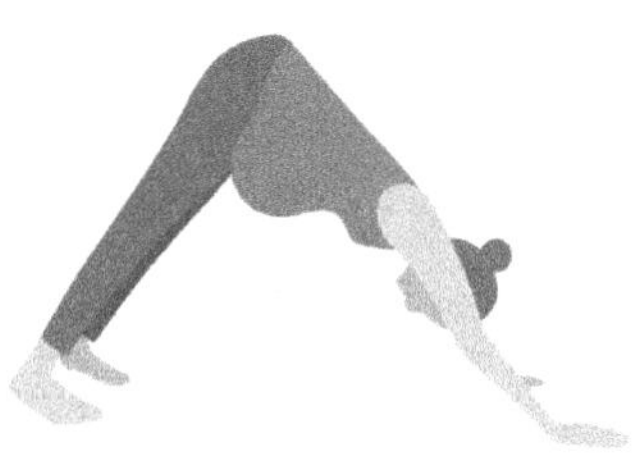

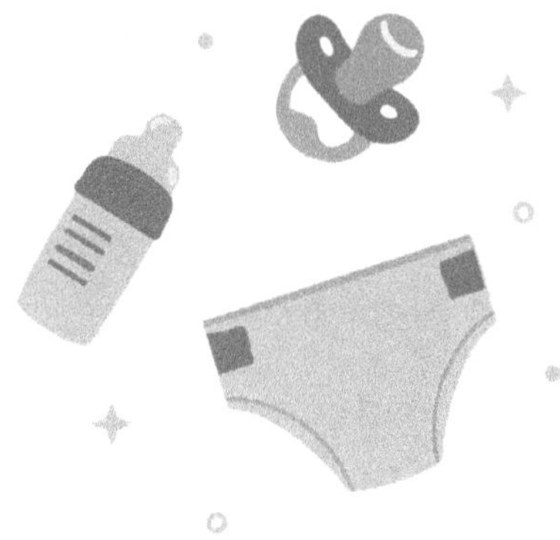

Prenatal Education and Classes

In this particular venture you're ready to start, the importance of prenatal education and classes cannot be overstated. Trust me; they can be a real lifesaver. Before I took those classes with Cláudia Boticas, the local Portuguese midwife, I had never even changed a diaper. I remember one instance when I had to look after a newborn while her mom went to the toilet. As luck would have it, the baby started crying inconsolably. In a panic, I tried to pacify her by shaking a toy, but it didn't work. The mom rushed out of the bathroom and told me the baby was just hungry. Clearly, I needed help. These classes were essential for everything from learning to establish a sleep routine to navigating basic tasks like installing a baby car seat and practicing breathing exercises. I can't stress enough how valuable my Portuguese midwife's guidance was to me.

I know you might not want to hear this, so let's get it over with quickly: Your baby can sense your anxiety. One of the best ways to feel more confident is by being prepared, and prenatal classes can help you with that. While the content of these classes can vary depending on where you are in the world, their aim is universal—to equip you with the knowledge and skills you need for a smoother pregnancy, labor, and postpartum experience. Plus, you get the added element of emotional support. You'll meet other expectant parents going through similar experiences, which could help you feel less anxious. You might even find a "bump buddy" or two. Involving your partner or a friend can make the experience even more enriching.

AVAILABILITY OF PRENATAL CLASSES IN DIFFERENT COUNTRIES

The registration process for prenatal classes can vary greatly from country to country. In Portugal, for example, my local general practitioner forwarded my details to the local midwife, who subsequently contacted me. Private options are available too, if you prefer a different program or teaching method. Perhaps an online course from your home country suits you better, or maybe your health insurance covers it. Whatever path you choose, make sure it's the right fit for you.

Here are some examples of how prenatal classes work in different countries:

United Kingdom

In the UK, the National Health Service (NHS) offers free antenatal classes to all pregnant women. These classes typically cover everything from labor and birth to breastfeeding and newborn care. Private options are also available if you prefer smaller groups or more specialized topics.

United States

In the US, prenatal classes are conducted widely through various channels such as hospitals, birthing centers, and private instructors. Options range from Lamaze and Bradley Method classes to hypnobirthing and water birth preparation. Many insurance plans cover the cost of these classes, so it's worth checking with your provider.

Australia

Australian healthcare systems provide extensive support for expectant mothers. The free or low-cost antenatal classes offered through public hospitals are particularly popular. These classes cover a range of topics including pain management, breastfeeding, and early parenting skills. Private classes are also available for those seeking more tailored support.

Japan

In Japan, prenatal classes are often offered through local health centers and maternity clinics. These classes emphasize natural childbirth and blend traditional practices with modern medical advice. Look for English-speaking options if needed.

Netherlands

The Netherlands is known for its comprehensive prenatal care, and prenatal classes are no exception. Classes are typically offered through midwives, hospitals, and private practitioners. They cover a range of topics including home birth preparation, which is common in the Netherlands.

Brazil

In Brazil, prenatal classes are offered through both public healthcare (SUS) and private healthcare providers. These classes often include discussions on pain relief options, breastfeeding, and postpartum care. Private classes may offer more personalized attention and flexible schedules.

Whether you're tackling the healthcare system in a new country or simply want to feel more prepared, attending local prenatal classes can be a game-changer. Embrace the opportunity to learn, connect, and prepare for the incredible adventure called parenthood.

TIPS ON FINDING PRENATAL CLASSES

• **Local Hospitals and Clinics**: Many hospitals and clinics offer prenatal classes. Check their websites or call their maternity departments to learn about their schedules and availability.

• **Community Centers**: Community centers often provide parenting and prenatal classes. Visit their websites or stop by to inquire about their offerings.

• **Online Platforms**: Websites like BabyCenter, The Bump, and even local Facebook groups can be great resources for finding both virtual and in-person classes.

• **Word of Mouth**: Ask friends, family, and/or colleagues, or pose a question to a social media group that's dedicated to people who have recently had babies. Personal recommendations can lead you to the best resources.

• **Doula Services**: Many doulas offer prenatal education as part of their services. Look for local doula associations or individual practitioners and sign up to seek the services of someone with whom you resonate.

• **Pediatrician or OB-GYN**: Your healthcare provider has the knowledge and resources to recommend reputable prenatal classes in your area. Don't hesitate to ask them for suggestions.

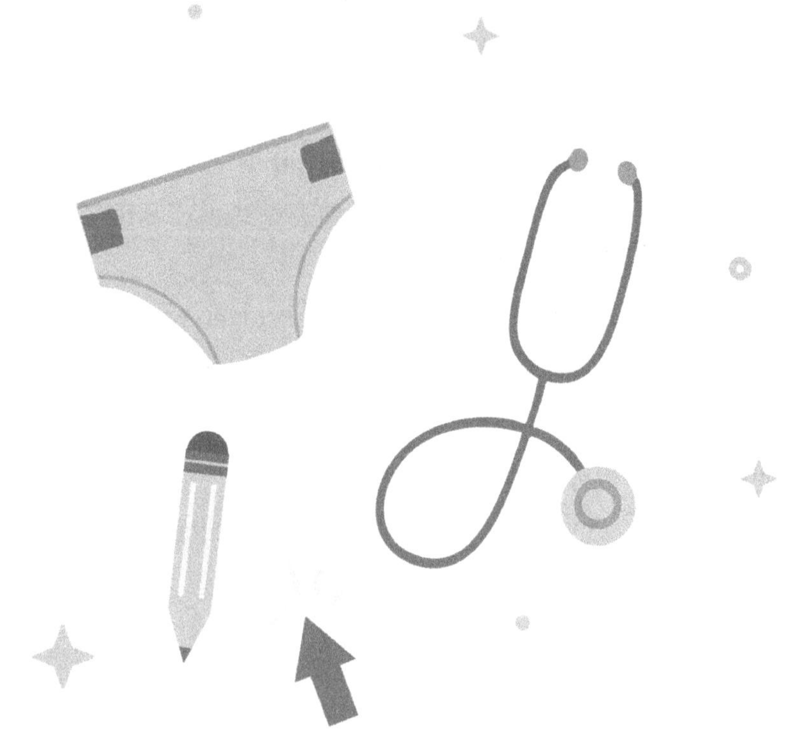

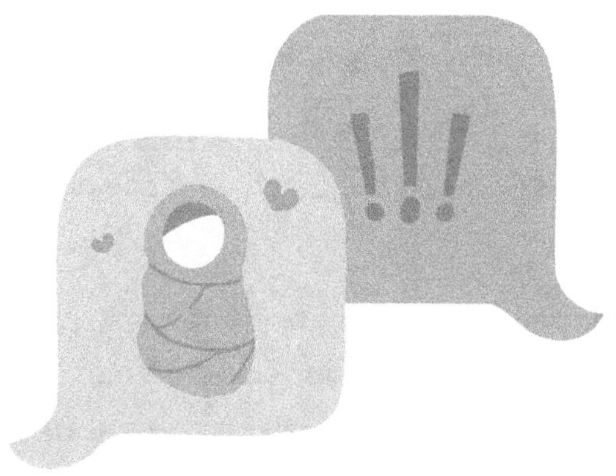

A Prenatal Care Experience in the Land Down Under: A Real-Life Tale

Luana pushed open the heavy glass doors of the hospital and stepped into the crisp afternoon air. She paused for a moment on the concrete steps, closed her eyes, and took a deep breath, hoping the fresh breeze would wash away the frustration gnawing at her.

This was her second baby, and although she knew what to expect from all the exams and procedures, she was still a little afraid. Her first birth experience had resulted in a second-degree laceration. Sure, it had healed, but the skin wasn't as strong as before. The fear of it (or something worse) happening again was very real. She needed that extra mental support and a lot of reassurance that everything would be okay.

During her appointment, the public doctor assigned to her had seemed more interested in ticking boxes on his clipboard than in connecting with her as a patient and addressing her concerns.

"Sit there," he had instructed curtly as soon as she entered the room, not once looking up at her. Instead, he was poring over his notebook.

Luana had barely settled before he directed her again, "Lie down." The brusqueness of his tone made her flinch, and the examination table was cold and uninviting.

She had hoped for some gentle encouragement, maybe a kind word or two. Instead, the doctor's actions were mechanical and devoid of any warmth. As he pressed the ultrasound wand to her belly, his eyes remained fixed on the screen, and she almost expected him to say, "Let's get this over with."

The entire appointment lasted less than fifteen minutes. He never enquired about how she was feeling or if she had any concerns. In fact, not once did he even smile at her. Once the checkup was completed, he handed her a printout of the scan and mumbled, "Next appointment in four weeks," before turning back to his desk.

Standing just outside the hospital doors, Luana clutched the ultrasound image in her hand and stared at the tiny blob that represented her baby. Despite knowing what to expect from the exams, she felt unsettled. Since she'd opted to go ahead with the public system, though, she didn't feel she had a choice but to accept the doctor who was assigned to her and brush the experience off. As she looked at the scanned image of her baby, her lips curved in a small smile. Despite the doctor's cold demeanor, this little life inside her was real. She already knew that she would do everything in her power to ensure a warm, supportive environment for her baby's arrival.

Although she'd never felt it necessary to use her husband's healthcare plan through his work, since she trusted the Australian public system, it finally came in handy. "I had a choice in private medicine. It felt great to know I could choose a doctor," she explained, and off she went on a search for her new doctor and a more compassionate path forward.

In the end, she recalls, "It was worth it. I felt secure and heard throughout the whole process."

The sun began to set, casting a golden hue over the city. As Luana gazed at the sky, she felt a renewed sense of purpose. This journey was just beginning, and she was determined to fill it with love and care, for both herself and her baby.

Luana's experience shows that the quality of prenatal care can vary significantly, not just because of the healthcare system but also due to individual doctors. For that reason, understanding and exploring your options is vital.

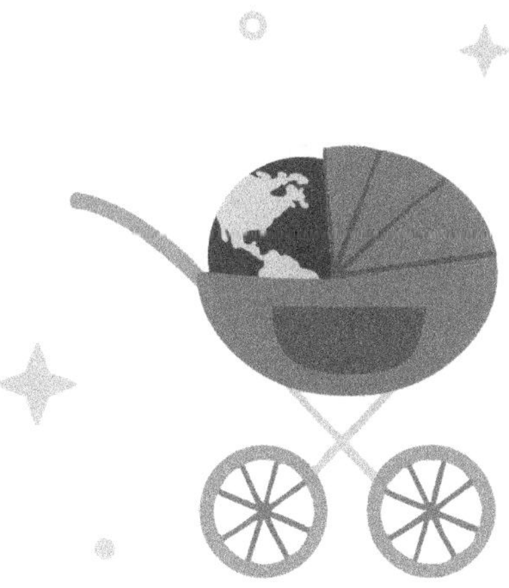

Summary of Key Points

UNDERSTANDING HEALTHCARE SYSTEMS

Understanding the healthcare system in your new country is a must—you need to know who provides the best care for a seamless, hassle-free experience.

• **Learn about the healthcare system in your new country.** You must understand how it works to access the care you need.

• **Get registered with a local doctor or clinic as soon as you arrive.** Don't wait until you need medical attention to find a healthcare provider.

• **Be prepared for emergencies by knowing local emergency numbers.** Keep these numbers handy in case you need them quickly.

• **Embrace local healthcare customs and be mindful of your budget.** Adapt to the local practices and manage your healthcare expenses wisely.

UNDERSTANDING PRENATAL CARE

• Figuring out prenatal care in a new country is essential for your (and your baby's!) well-being. However, their system may be highly nuanced, which is why it is important to do your research.

• **Learn the Basics of Prenatal Care:** Understanding the essentials of prenatal care—regardless of where you're living—will help you advocate for yourself and keep you and your baby healthy. Regular checkups and prenatal testing are imperative for early detection and treatment of potential health issues.

- **Set up Your Prenatal Visits**: As soon as you settle in, register with a local doctor or a midwife. They'll set up a schedule for your prenatal visits, which will become more frequent as your due date approaches, especially if you're over 35 or have a high-risk pregnancy.

- **Referrals and Appointments**: Your access to prenatal services can vary greatly depending on the healthcare system where you are. In some places, you might need a referral from a general practitioner to see an obstetrician, while in others, you can go directly to a specialist. Understanding these protocols will save you time and stress. Make sure to find a reliable general practitioner early on to avoid delays in your prenatal care.

- **Maintain a Balanced Diet**: Look for nutrient-rich foods and adapt your meals to include essential nutrients like folic acid, iron, calcium, and DHA. Embrace local dietary recommendations and consult with local nutritionists or healthcare providers for tailored advice.

- **Find Familiar Foods and Adapt Recipes**: Craving familiar foods? Look for international grocery stores or shop online. Have fun exploring local markets, where you'll discover fresh produce and local delicacies. Try putting a local twist on your favorite recipes to blend the familiar with the new.

- **Stay Active During Pregnancy**: Staying active is vital. Join local prenatal exercise classes, explore outdoor activities, and adapt to the climate. Whether it's yoga, walking, or gentle hikes, find activities that keep you moving.

- **Prenatal Education and Classes**: Enroll in prenatal classes to gain valuable knowledge. The people you meet there often extend invaluable emotional support. These classes vary from country to country but aim to prepare you for pregnancy, labor, and postpartum matters. Meeting other expectant parents can also provide a supportive community.

By following these key points, you'll be better prepared to manage prenatal care in your new country, ensuring a healthier and more enjoyable journey for both you and your baby.

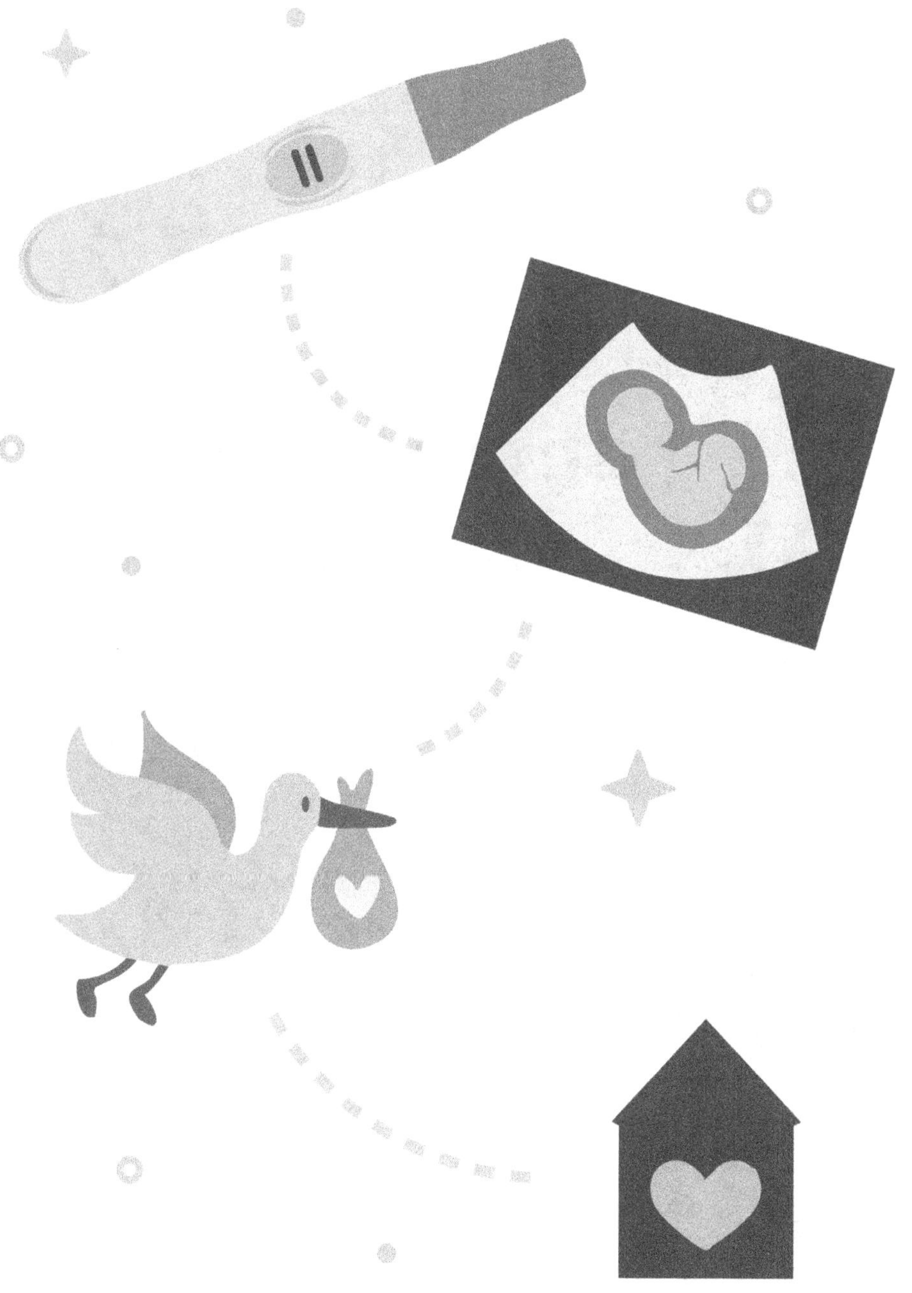

PART 2

Establishing A Strong Foundation: Health Insurance, Legalities, And A Support Network

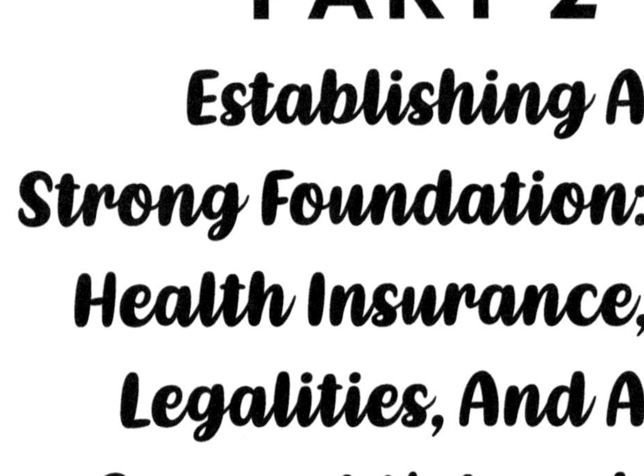

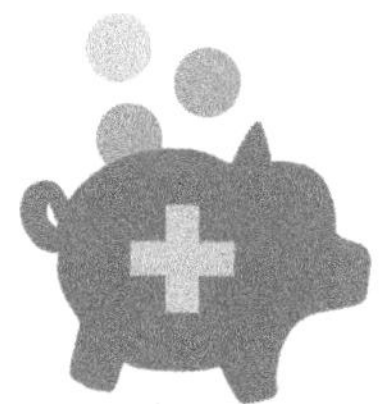

Figuring out the details of **health insurance, legalities, and parental leave** in a new country can be as confusing as trying to understand why Pumpkin Spice Lattes have such a cult following—everyone seems to love them, but you don't really get it until you try one! So, what's covered? What isn't? What should you look for in the fine print? Let's unravel the tangle of this insurance knot together, one thread at a time, and explore how to create a **supportive community** while you're away from your native land and possibly your family.

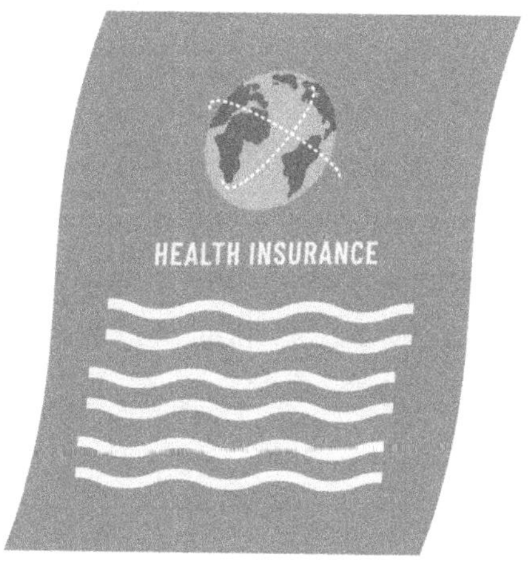

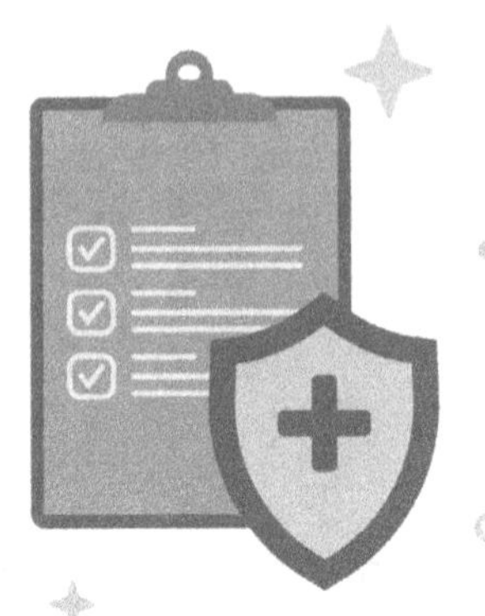

HEALTH INSURANCE

When setting up your life in a new country, you need to understand the type of health insurance that best fits your needs. So, let's dive into the two main types of health insurance: international and local. In particular, let's explore the specific situations they are each designed to address.

INTERNATIONAL HEALTH INSURANCE: YOUR GLOBAL SAFETY NET

Imagine you're a frequent traveler or someone who hasn't decided where to settle down yet. If you move frequently between countries or travel often for work or leisure, managing healthcare can be especially challenging. How can you stay safe and healthy miles away from home? This is where international health insurance comes to your rescue. Think of it as a global safety net, designed to provide extensive healthcare coverage across multiple countries, which is essential if you:

- Move frequently between countries

- Travel often for work or leisure

- Seek consistent access to healthcare standards similar to those in your home country

While there's no one-size-fits-all "global insurance," some plans are designed for frequent travelers and allow them to enjoy healthcare standards similar to those in their home country at all times.

In fact, many international health insurance providers offer policies that cater to expatriates and frequent travelers. These plans often cover a wide range of countries, allowing you access to healthcare services no matter where you are. They also typically provide comprehensive coverage, including a broad network of healthcare providers around the world and even emergency evacuation when necessary.

These plans can be a lifesaver for those who don't stick to one place for too long and need reliable healthcare wherever they go. Especially when you're pregnant, traveling extensively can be quite difficult. Thankfully, having a healthcare plan that accounts for your frequent traveling can provide peace of mind and ensure you and your baby are always cared for, no matter where your journeys take you.

BENEFITS OF INTERNATIONAL HEALTH INSURANCE

- **Consistent Coverage:** You can avoid the hassle of switching plans if you move to another country, ensuring continuity in prenatal healthcare or treatment for ongoing health issues.

- **Broader Medical Access:** International health insurance provides access to a wider network of doctors and hospitals.

Often, these plans also allow people to seek treatment in facilities that either cater specifically to foreigners or offer services similar to those in the Western world.

- **Emergency Evacuation:** Emergency evacuation is included in many international plans, which can be a lifesaver if you're in a remote or less-developed area where adequate medical facilities are not available.

LOCAL HEALTH INSURANCE: TAILORED TO YOUR IMMEDIATE ENVIRONMENT

While international health insurance plans offer many advantages, local health insurance is more suitable if you're planning to stay in one country for an extended period. It's typically less expensive than international insurance but is tailored to the healthcare system of the country in which you're living. This type of insurance is perfect if you:

- Have a permanent residence in a specific country or are planning to stay in the same place for the foreseeable future

- Prefer using local healthcare services

- Need coverage that aligns closely with local legal and medical standards

CONSIDERATIONS FOR LOCAL HEALTH INSURANCE

- **Cost-Effectiveness:** Typically, these plans come with lower premiums than international insurance, making them more budget-friendly. So, it may be a better option for those who don't frequently travel internationally. **Localized Service:** Since providers are usually very familiar with the local healthcare system, you can expect faster and more effective treatment.

- **Limitations on Coverage:** Coverage is limited to the host country. So, if you have plans to visit your home country frequently, this plan might be inconvenient. The cost benefit quickly comes down with this option if you need coverage across multiple countries, as they can get more expensive.

CHOOSING BETWEEN INTERNATIONAL AND LOCAL INSURANCE

Since both categories of health insurance plans come with their own set of advantages, your lifestyle and medical needs can help you pick the right type for you. If you haven't permanently settled in a country yet, or if you enjoy living an international lifestyle, international health insurance offers a flexible and comprehensive solution. However, if your life is firmly rooted in one location, local health insurance can provide tailored and cost-effective coverage.

Remember, whether you choose local or international health insurance plans, your location plays a big role in the overall cost of your package. The price may also depend on quite a lot of factors like your age, health status, and coverage levels. In fact, it is very interesting to note that private healthcare costs can vary dramatically between countries, even those that are geographically close. Your international health insurance premium will reflect these differences. For example, in 2023, the average annual cost of health insurance in Singapore was a whopping $7,764. That's nearly double what you'd pay in Vietnam, where expat health insurance averages around $3,934 annually.[6]

And if you think that's high, check this out: the USA tops the list at $9,817 per year, followed by Hong Kong at $7,810. Dubai isn't much cheaper, at $5,687 annually![6] As you can see, where you live can make a huge difference in how much you pay for health coverage.

In terms of local health insurance, the annual premiums for domestic policies can range from $300 to $1,200 per year in countries with public healthcare systems.[6]

Remember, it's a good idea to consider your personal circumstances, including your health status, mobility, and financial flexibility before making a choice. The best way to make an informed decision is by doing your own research or requesting the help of an insurance advisor, since these approaches can provide important personalized insights.[6]

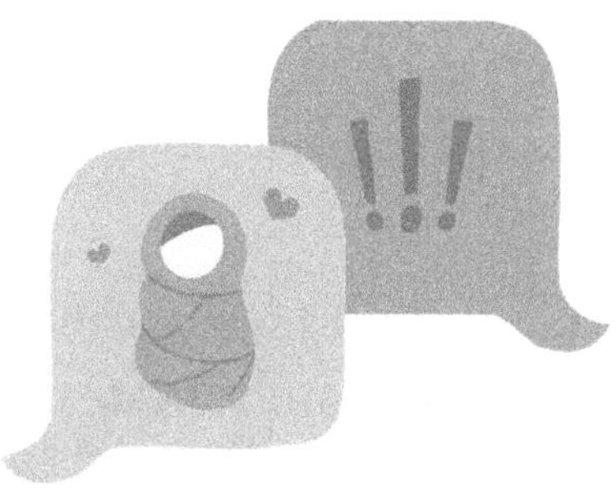

Navigating the Insurance Labyrinth: My Own Real-Life Tale

Honestly, I don't know what I was thinking when I shrugged off the more expensive options with a naive, "Why would I need that?" mentality and instead signed up for what seemed like reasonably-priced health insurance. Based on my experience, let me tell you this—always plan ahead, especially when you're about to start a family and have a history of health issues like endometriosis.

I moved to Portugal from Ireland with a diagnosis of two giant ovarian cysts and endometriosis. I tried to get in touch with a local public general practitioner and was stunned to learn that no slots were available for a whole year. I felt caught between a rock and a hard place, and I had no choice but to explore the private option. So, when Dr. Ana Sofia Fernandes in Portugal offered me a quicker private possibility, I jumped at it without thinking twice. She wasn't just any doctor; she was a fertility specialist and obstetrician—a true fairy godmother who offered me a real solution.

The surgery set me back about $10,000, which was a huge financial hit. I learned the hard way that 70% coverage doesn't mean much when you're not clear on the fine print. And as for discounts on related costs like electricity during hospital stays (yes, that was a thing) ... there were none.

Fast forward a few months, and I was pregnant, thanks to the excellent care I received. But I chose to stick with private care, unwilling to risk not having Dr. Ana Sofia Fernandes deliver my baby. The childbirth alone cost another $5,000. Again, it was more than I had anticipated.

Only after these expenses did I seriously reconsider my insurance choices. Unfortunately, by then it was too late to switch plans without facing long waiting periods, and I was already deep into this brand-new territory where I needed medical help constantly. I had to stick with my current plan, which meant no clear cost estimates and potential additional charges if complications arose.

It's not like the baby we wasn't planned! I blame myself, really. I should have dug deeper into the fine print and learned more. When I signed up for the insurance plan, I didn't consider that I might want to go through a specific private doctor and hospital, which some insurances covered but others did not. Could I have chosen to go public? Absolutely. In fact, I did choose to do my prenatal course through the public system because it was great. But I decided to go private, despite the hefty bills, because I wanted to go through this experience with the doctor I felt connected to—the one who, right after my endometriosis surgery, had a sunny smile on her face telling me everything went well. I wanted the certainty of her presence throughout the pregnancy and after delivery, and that decision added a lot of unexpected pressure and anxiety.

Looking back, I wish I'd paid more attention to the details of my health insurance plan from the start. It's key, especially as an immigrant, to understand exactly what you're signing up for and to anticipate future health needs as much as possible. I discovered firsthand that being prepared isn't simply about having any insurance—it's about having the right insurance for your life's unpredictable twists and turns.

For example, my plan covered a good amount in a different hospital but not in the one I needed, and I didn't take that fact into account. I had to pay to cover the room, my husband's accommodation, food for the two of us, extras like exams for the baby, and medication ... in addition to the fee for the doctor, the anesthetist, and the nurses. And we paid a COVID fee too.

So, if you're moving abroad or considering a new health insurance plan, please take my advice. Read the fine print, plan for the unexpected, and maybe, just maybe, consider the pricier option if it means better coverage. It might just save you a lot of headaches and heartaches down the road.

Legalities And Leaves

Since we're now sorted in terms of pre- and post-natal healthcare, it's time to get into a few more important topics. Dealing with **birthright citizenship**, **parental leave**, and **paperwork** in a new country can be like trying to ask for directions when you don't speak the language—you think you're getting somewhere, but you might just end up more lost! Each country has its own wild mix of laws—about who gets to be a citizen and how long you can chill at home with your new baby—that can make your head spin.

So, let's dive into these legal mazes, armed with some real-life stories, and figure out how to tackle this issue like a pro. Grab your drink of choice, and let's decode these puzzles together, shall we?

Birthright Citizenship

Did you know every country has its own rules about granting citizenship to newborns? Where your child is born could drastically impact whether they're considered a citizen of that country, your home country, or even both.

HERE'S THE SCOOP ON GLOBAL CITIZENSHIP LAWS

If you're living abroad or planning to have a baby in another country, getting a handle on both your host and home country's citizenship laws is super important, as it can affect your child's future in big ways.

Jus Soli (Right of the Soil)

Take the U.S. and Canada, for example. If your baby is born on either of these countries' soil, boom! They automatically get citizenship. Just like that. Alessandra Ravasi's daughter, Paula, was born in North Virginia and got her U.S. citizenship at birth. But Alessandra's son, born back in Brazil, had to wait until his parents were recognized as citizens. Isn't it fascinating how these laws work?

Jus Sanguinis (Right of Blood)

Now, flipping over to places like Europe and Australia, it's interesting to note that they follow a different beat with *jus sanguinis*, meaning "right of blood." This principle means the baby's citizenship depends on their parents' citizenships instead of where they're born. For instance,

Gaby was born in Brisbane to a Brazilian mother on a visa. She didn't get Australian citizenship but became a citizen of New Zealand through her father and a Brazilian citizen through her mother.

WHEN THINGS GET COMPLICATED

Dual or Multiple Citizenship Example

If you're born in a country that doesn't allow dual nationality, you need to make some tough calls. Take Tomo, for example. He was born in Japan but then moved to Australia. To become an Australian citizen, he would have had to give up his Japanese citizenship, but he chose not to. A lot of foreigners face this tough decision, and some prefer to stay on a permanent visa to avoid losing their original nationality.

In Australia, Tomo met Fabiola Imamura, a Brazilian who got her Australian citizenship after living there for several years. Thanks to Australia's laws, she could enjoy the benefits of dual nationality. Nine years ago, they had a son together and named him Jake. So, what are Jake's citizenship options? Lucky Jake gets all three! Brazil and Australia are cool with dual (or even triple) citizenship. Jake is an Aussie because he was born there; he can claim Brazilian citizenship through his mom; and he has Japanese citizenship because Japan allows kids born to Japanese parents to claim multiple nationalities until they turn 22.

Jake hit the jackpot with citizenships, thanks to his parents' diverse backgrounds!

THE UPSIDES OF DUAL CITIZENSHIP

So, what does this citizenship smorgasbord mean for Jake? Well, dual citizenship comes with a bunch of perks:

- **Education and Healthcare**: Jake can access schools and hospitals in all three countries. Imagine having the choice of universities across continents or being able to get healthcare wherever you are!

- **Travel Freedom**: Jake can be a passport-holder in all three countries. This privilege means fewer visa hassles and more freedom to explore the world.

- **Job Opportunities**: Holding multiple citizenships opens up job markets in all three countries. Jake can choose where he wants to work without worrying about work permits.

THE NOT-SO-GREAT PARTS

But it's not all sunshine and rainbows. Dual citizenship has its challenges too:

- **Legal Obligations**: Jake might have to deal with all three countries' tax laws. This scenario can get a bit complicated, and he might require some professional help to avoid costly errors.

- **Military Service**: Some countries require their citizens to do military service, so Jake could be on the hook for that in any of his countries.

- **Cultural Juggling**: Balancing multiple cultural identities can be tricky. Jake might find it challenging to understand and appreciate his diverse heritage.

So, dual citizenship is a mixed bag of amazing opportunities and some potential headaches. For kids like Jake, it means a world full of options and responsibilities. With a bit of preparation and understanding, they can make the most of their unique situation.

WHEN CITIZENSHIP GETS OVERTURNED BY ANOTHER LAW

When Larissa went to the UK before the pandemic, she wasn't married to Guy yet, but she was already pregnant with their child. That's when she learned that, legally, the baby was solely hers. In other words, she had complete parental responsibility. "Luke was mine, and I had total authority," she explains. According to the UK government's official website, all mothers automatically have parental responsibility. Fathers only enjoy this responsibility if they're married to the mother or listed on the birth certificate.[7]

"If I hadn't married and instead decided to jet off, he [the father] couldn't have done a thing about it," she laughs. Luckily, this beautiful family chose to become even more united. Had they decided not to marry each other, it could have impacted Luke's citizenship options. This scenario shows how complex things can get when different countries' laws affect family decisions.

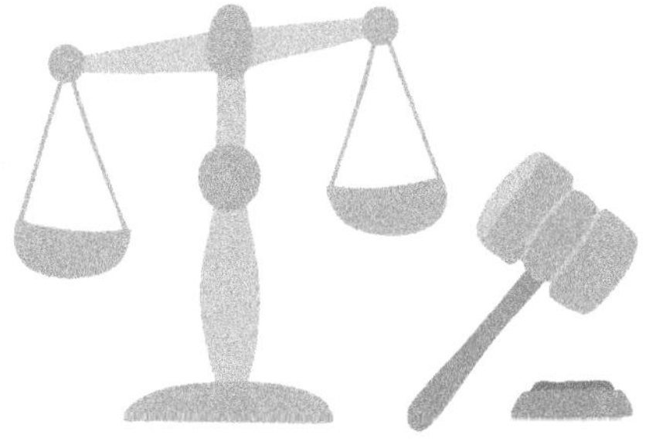

Navigating These Tricky Waters

Getting your head around all these rules is very important, especially when you're living life abroad. If you still need further help, here's what you can do:

- **Chat with a lawyer** who knows their stuff about citizenship and family law.

- **Don't hesitate to hit up your embassy** if you need clarity or help figuring out your child's legal status.

- **Look online for resources and forums** where other expats share their experiences and advice. Plenty of websites and communities are dedicated to helping you comprehend these issues.

Understanding these complex legal landscapes ensures your child gets the right citizenship, which paves the way for their future opportunities. And trust me, getting this sorted out can really put your mind at ease. So, sip that coffee and start untangling those legal knots—it's worth the effort!

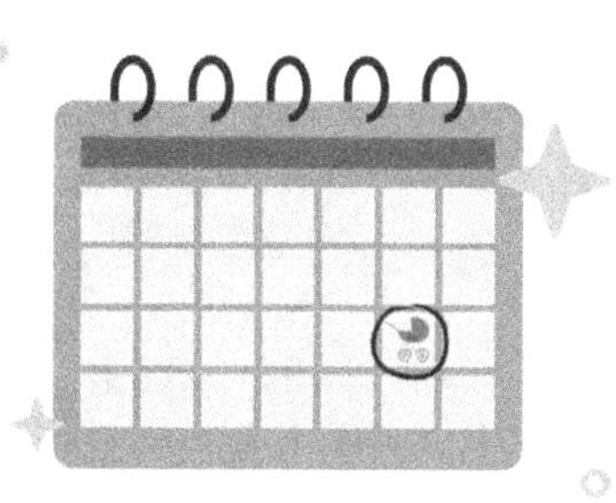

PARENTAL LEAVE

Figuring out parental leave in a new country is key to learning how to balance new careers and family life in completely unfamiliar territory. This is especially true if you're traveling for work, as it adds an extra layer of complexity when you're trying to achieve that perfect balance.

A QUICK WORLD TOUR OF PARENTAL LEAVE

So, parental leave is the time you get off of work to hang out and bond with your new kiddo, right? The thing is it can look way different depending on where you are:

- **Bulgaria** goes all out with 410 days of leave. More importantly, you get 90% of your salary during this leave. Then, they keep the support coming until your little one turns two.[9]

- **Norway** lets you choose between two great options. You can either take 59 weeks off at 80% pay or 49 weeks with your full salary.

Dads get a sweet deal too, with up to 10 weeks available depending on what their partner earns. [9]

- In **Sweden**, parents get a whopping 480 days of leave paid at 80%, and they can split it however they like. Multiple births? No problem, they give you extra time for that too.[9]

- **Germany** gives you 14 weeks fully-paid leave right off the bat, and then you can decide to stay home for up to three years to bond with your baby.[9] During parental leave, the parent "will not receive a salary from your employer. However, you can apply for parental allowance, a form of financial support from the government that compensates you if you temporarily work less or not at all after the birth of your child."[8]

- **Greece** offers up to 43 weeks of leave. While you receive full pay for the first 17 weeks, your pay then drops to minimum wage for six more months. Plus, you can work fewer hours when you return to work.[9]

- And then there's **Japan**, which is setting the pace for dads with up to 12 months of paternity leave.

- **Iceland** splits six months of leave equally between both parents. [9]

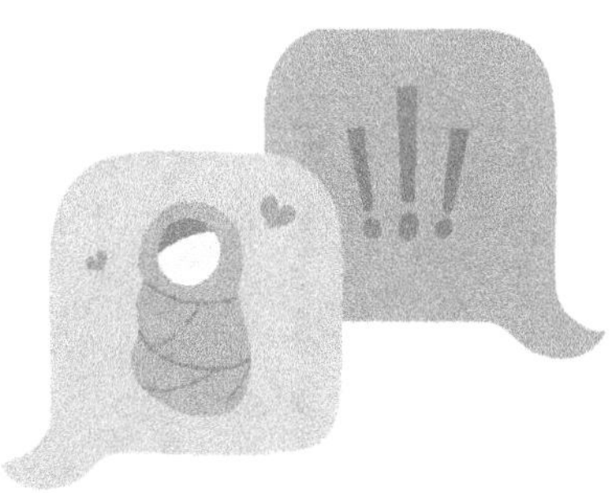

Amanda's Unimaginable Parental Leave Benefits: A Real-Life Tale

In 2017, Amanda Santos couldn't hold back her giggle any longer as she sat in front of the government employee who dealt with parental leave policy implementation. She never imagined she'd hear, "You can take up to three years of parental leave. How many years do you want?" It felt like a prank. In Brazil, the standard is just 120 days! How could maternity leave be so long? "I thought it was absurd ... bizarre even. I said 'one year' immediately, and then I realized that one year was too short."

Amanda quickly learned about the benefits of Austria's parental leave policy. "I think they were paying around 580 euros per month, and you could work 20 hours within that period too. You couldn't work full-time. But once the child was one or one-and-a-half years old and could go to daycare, you could work some hours and still receive the payment. I found that incredible, and the social system here works very well.

"A year felt too short without my mom, relatives, or anyone to help. I did everything with Ana. I went to the bathroom with Ana, the doctor with Ana, shopping with Ana. I didn't leave her alone for a minute because I was alone with her. My husband helped a lot when he came home from work. He'd say, 'Go sleep,' and at 9 or 10 p.m., I'd wake up and take over."

Amanda appreciated that the policy allowed her to balance work and childcare. And when it was time to welcome her second child, Amanda opted for a longer break. She found that extra time really helped her and her baby adjust slowly and gave them more space to bond as a family.

Why All This Matters

These differences aren't just about time off; they tell us a lot about what each country values:

- **Gender Equality:** Places like Sweden and Japan are at the very top when it comes to making sure dads get time off too. Their policies help challenge old-school gender roles and make it easier for moms to get back to work.

- **Economic Effects:** In Norway and Sweden, strong parental leave policies mean people stick with their jobs longer, which is great for businesses and the economy.

- **Better Health for Kids and Parents:** More time with your baby can mean better breastfeeding percentages, timely vaccinations, and improved bonding, all of which can be challenging for some mothers.

- **Cultural Insights:** How a country handles parental leave truly reflects its cultural values. Bulgaria's lengthy leave demonstrates a strong emphasis on family care, while the varied parental leave policies across different companies in the U.S. highlight that country's diverse views on work-life balance.

- **Changing Trends:** Watching how countries change their rules about parental leave, such as Iceland and Japan extending paternity leave, shows shifting views on parenting roles.

TIPS FOR FOREIGNERS

Getting to know these policies and following them goes well beyond the logistics; it's about really getting into the cultural swing of your new home. Knowing the ins and outs can make a huge difference and can help you thrive in your new environment instead of merely surviving. Chat with a lawyer, hit up your embassy, and definitely talk to other people who have gone through it. Plenty of online forums also offer advice and support from those in your boat.

So, as we sip our decaf coffee and think about all this (I need double the caffeine, though, because my 18-month-old is teething six teeth at once, and most of them are the big back ones—*send help!*), remember that understanding parental leave abroad is crucial for making your time there a smashing success.

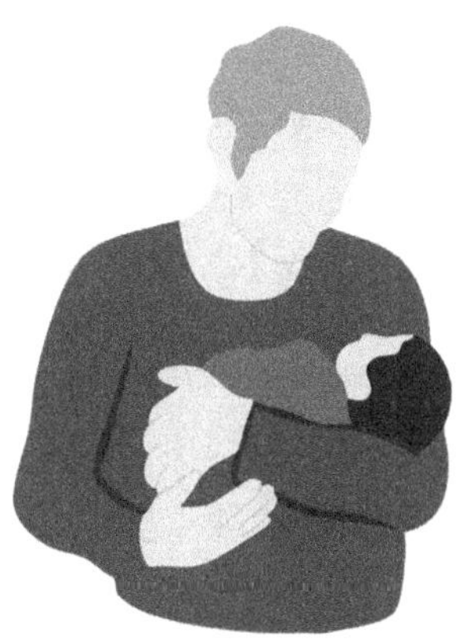

PAPERWORK

Bringing home a new baby is a joyous occasion, but it also means you've got to tackle a pile of paperwork that can be just as exhausting as those sleepless nights. Especially if you're living abroad, figuring out how to register the birth and get the right citizenship documents in your host country can be challenging.

Take Flávia, for example. Living in Okinawa, she found herself in quite a pickle when trying to register her daughter's Brazilian citizenship. "It's a whole bureaucratic tangle," she tells me. Without a Brazilian consulate on the island, she'd need to catch a flight to Tokyo or Nagoya to begin the paperwork. Each of these places is a hefty two-and-a-half hours away. "For now, she's essentially without a nationality," Flávia sighs, evidence of how stressful things can be during what should be a happy time.

Flávia's ordeal really drives home why it's so important to get a jump on this stuff. If you're a foreign parent, here's a handy guide that will hopefully prevent you from getting bogged down:

- **Early Contact:** Hit up your home country's embassy or consulate ASAP to get the lowdown on what paperwork you'll need and how long it'll take.

- **Plan for Travel:** Stuck in a place without easy consular access? Better start thinking about where you can go to sort out the necessary documents. A trip may be necessary to get all of this sorted.

- **Seek Local Advice:** Tap into local expat communities or parenting groups. These are great places to get tips and tricks from others who have already gone through it.

- **Prepare Documents:** Proactively round up all the documents you might need. We're talking passports, visa details, marriage certificates, and proof of residency.

- **Legal Advice:** Sometimes, it's wise to chat with a legal advisor who's clued in to both your host and your home country's laws about citizenship and parental rights.

By getting ahead of these tasks, you can cut down on the bureaucratic headaches and spend more time enjoying your new bundle of joy. Being prepared is paramount, as it ensures that your little one's legal identity and rights are set up right, no matter where in the world you find yourselves.

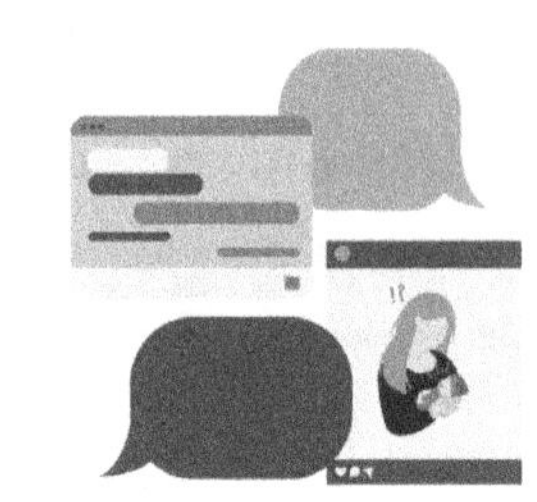

BUILDING A SUPPORT NETWORK

Adjusting to life in a new country can definitely throw you some curveballs, especially when you're starting or raising a family there. One of the most important things you can do to make this transition smoother is to build a solid support network. I'm not just talking about making friends, though that's important too! I'm talking about a network that will serve as your lifeline, offering emotional, practical, and informational support to keep you steady in unfamiliar waters. In the following sections, I'll share some suggestions about who to include in your support network, from healthcare providers to fellow expat parents who can help you manage this new chapter with confidence.

YOUR HEALTHCARE HERO: FINDING THE ONE

When you move to a new country, finding the right healthcare provider is as important as finding a place to live. Beyond treating an illness, it's about finding someone who really understands you, speaks your language both literally and figuratively, and gets the unique challenges you face as a transplant in new soil.

Take Debora Cunha, a Brazilian immigrant living in Queenstown, New Zealand, for example. She emphasizes how imperative it is to choose the right doctor. "For me, it was crucial because I was initially afraid of hospitals," she explains. "Building a trustful relationship with my doctor helped alleviate my fears." That kind of bond with your healthcare provider becomes a cornerstone of comfort and security in your new world.

Language barriers can make navigating healthcare a bit tricky, but Alessandra Ravasi, living in Northern Virginia, found a way to turn this challenge into a positive experience. She made sure to choose a doctor who spoke her language—Portuguese. "My doctor was Argentinian-American, so we had plenty of options," she shares with a smile. Interestingly, even with all those language choices, Alessandra opted to speak English during her appointments. "I wanted to be ready for anything," she says, making sure she could handle the local medical scene like a pro.

Sometimes, the key to finding the right healthcare professional is tapping into your new community. Danielle Rocha, who moved in 2016 from Brazil to Miami, is a testament to this idea. "I had many insecurities as a first-time mother in another country. The way I found to feel safe was to look for information. So, I got a pregnancy book, you know? And then I said, 'Wow, I'm full of doubts.' The great support resource at the time was an instant messaging group of the women from my husband's work. One of them had recently had a baby and recommended her doctor, an American Cuban, who had a warm, human touch. I loved him. At the consultation, he kissed me on the cheek, helped me get off the table, and just made all these little gestures that made me feel safer. He also gave me space to ask questions via email. I was totally crazy, sending a list of questions every week, and he answered everything."

When searching for your healthcare hero, certain considerations are very important. While their professional credentials certainly matter, you should also look at their ability to communicate effectively in a language you're comfortable with, their experience with patients from different cultural backgrounds, what other expatriates say about them, and how convenient their office location is.

Finding the right healthcare provider is a critical step in settling into a new country. It can be challenging, but it's also an opportunity to connect with your new community and ensure that your health needs are met with understanding and care.

CHECKLIST FOR FINDING A HEALTHCARE PROVIDER

☑ Ask for recommendations from friends, neighbors, and expat communities.

☑ Use online resources to find and review potential doctors.

☑ Verify the doctor's qualifications and language proficiency.

☑ Prepare questions for your initial consultation.

☑ Bring your medical records to the first visit.

☑ Assess your comfort level with the doctor and the clinic environment.

☑ Join expat and healthcare support groups for additional advice and community support. You can usually find these groups online through social media platforms, forums, and dedicated websites. Additionally, many local communities offer in-person support groups and meetups, which can be a great way to connect with others in similar situations.

By following these steps and joining support groups, you'll be well able to properly meet your health needs in your new home. This approach will help you build a strong foundation for your life abroad and help you feel safe and well-cared for in your new community.

EXPATRIATE GROUPS

Groups for expatriates are integral for anyone trying to settle into life in a new country, especially during big life changes like becoming a parent. They're so much more than a way to meet people; they're a lifeline. They provide the much-needed sense of community that can be hard to find so far from home.

Alana, who currently lives in Amsterdam, shared just how important such a group was for her. "Back in Brazil, none of my friends were having kids; I had no family around, so I was building all this knowledge from scratch. I only had one friend here, and she was dealing with her own new baby, so she couldn't offer much help. That's when I realized I needed to branch out and build my support network. Here, they have tons of WhatsApp groups," she said. "It's 3 a.m., my baby's crying with a fever, and I'm freaking out. I message the group, and instantly, I have lots of moms giving me advice. It's this invisible, yet visible support network. I don't know these people personally, but they're there, even at three in the morning, helping me figure out what to do. It's amazing."

Joining a group for newcomers like yourself can really smooth out the rough edges of moving to a new place and settling in there. These communities are great for giving practical advice. Whether it's finding top-notch local healthcare or understanding cultural quirks and bureaucratic situations, such support groups go a long way in helping you feel at home in a new country. But more importantly, they offer emotional support through shared experiences. They're about swapping stories, laughing over cultural mix-ups, and getting tips on how to handle homesickness. The value of connecting with someone who just 'gets it' is immeasurable.

Many groups (both local and those meant for expats) don't stop online; they organize regular meetups, language exchanges, and family-friendly events that can spice up your social life and help you build lasting friendships. For foreign parents, these groups often organize playdates, mom and baby mornings, and even parenting workshops. It's a great way to feel like part of a community, since it's is normal to experience loneliness and isolation as a parent in a foreign country.

And let's not overlook the power of today's digital age. Platforms like Facebook, Instagram, Reddit, and other social media groups provide around-the-clock access to community advice and support. Whether you're dealing with an emergency, looking for a local service, or just need to vent after a tough day, someone is almost always in the same time zone—or even just around the corner—who can lend a hand or an ear. Alana adds, "Look for your support network; find WhatsApp groups. I have like fifteen groups! No matter what phase you're going through, a resource is out there to help you, including groups for food introduction, groups for expectant moms, groups for the elderly, expat groups, neighborhood walking groups, and so much more. It's an amazing network that has grown around these needs. Foreign life can be really lonely, so we need to support each other in this journey."

Expat groups provide a platform for connection and camaraderie that can make living abroad feel a bit more like home. They remind us that, while we might be far from our native lands, we're not alone. These groups can be incredibly helpful in understanding and dealing with the bureaucratic aspects of living in a new country. They can help you work with documentation requirements and understand local regulations better.

So, if you ever find yourself feeling overwhelmed by the foreign experience, remember that an expat group is more than likely waiting to welcome you with open arms. These friends often become the chosen family we rely on for both emotional and practical support during the most transformative periods of our lives.

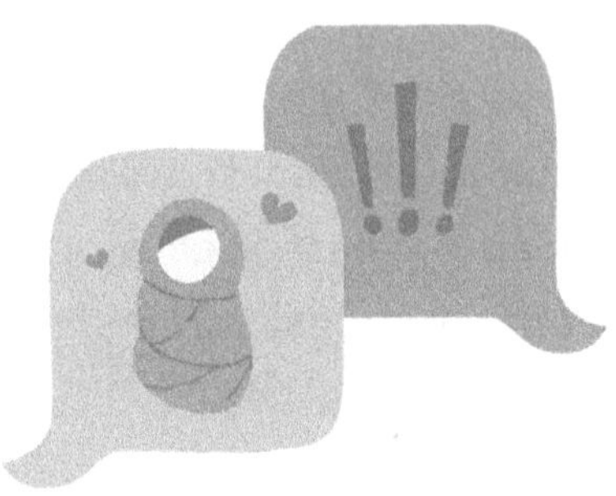

Maria's Real-Life Tale:
Finding Light in the Darkest of Times

In 2014, just before the Carnival season, Brazil buzzed with warm weather and vibrant parties. In Bahia, Maria Heneghan's home state, celebrations were inescapable, with confetti finding its way into every corner. But that year, Maria felt different, as she had just moved to Australia from Brazil with her four-month-old son. While she watched the festivities from afar, her new reality of caring for her baby full-time made her feel a world away from the vibrant celebrations she once knew.

"I remember it as if it were today," she recalls. One gloomy evening, feeling overwhelmed and close to giving up on her new home, Maria stared at her computer keyboard. "What if...?" she wondered, but quickly dismissed the thought, fearing it was foolish. "Who would even read what I have to say?" her inner critic whispered. But the persistent ache of loneliness wouldn't let go. Having just arrived in Brisbane, she had no friends, and her husband, whom she loved dearly, travelled frequently for work. "My English was terrible," she recalls. "I felt isolated, taking care of our child alone."

Maria never thought her quest for adventure and language learning in Ireland would take this turn. She met her other half in Europe, but when she got pregnant, complications forced her to return to Brazil for the birth. Months later, the new family reunited in Australia because of her husband's work relocation. Because of this sudden migration with a newborn, she found it hard to build a social life and became depressed.

Desperate for some friendly connection, Maria turned to a local Facebook group for Brazilian expatriates. "I opened my heart," she says. "I posted about my loneliness and struggles and called for other mothers to meet in person."

The response was overwhelming. Encouraged, Maria organized a picnic, and 70 mothers showed up. That day marked a turning point. Since then, she took it upon herself to create opportunities and events that would take this connection to another level. She organized playdates, parties, and dance classes, each of which strengthened the community bonds. Now, Maria feels a profound sense of belonging. By sharing her story, she transformed her darkest times into a life filled with light and laughter and even created a safe space for other struggling mothers.

Maria's story beautifully illustrates the transformative power of building a support network. Just as she found light in the darkest of times by connecting with others, you too can face the challenges of foreign life by creating a strong support system. Whether it's through finding your healthcare hero, joining expatriate groups, or simply reaching out for help when you need it, these connections can turn isolation into community, uncertainty into confidence, and challenges into triumphs. So, as you embark on your venture of maternity abroad, remember that you're not alone. A world of support is waiting for you.

Summary of Key Points

NAVIGATING HEALTH INSURANCE

Choosing health insurance can be challenging, so understanding your options is key:

1. **Understand the Differences:** Learn about the differences between international and local health insurance plans to figure out how they suit your specific needs.

2. **Evaluate Your Needs:** Consider factors like cost, coverage, and your personal health requirements when selecting a plan.

3. **Consult an Expert:** Speak with an insurance advisor to make an informed decision. This way, you can be sure the plan suits your circumstances.

LEGALITIES AND PARENTAL LEAVE

1. **Learn the Basics:** Familiarize yourself with your host or home country's citizenship laws. Know who is eligible and what benefits apply.

2. **Evaluate Parental Leave Policies**: Understand the parental leave policies and how they can benefit you. How much time can you take off and what exactly are you entitled to?

3. **Seek Professional Guidance**: Consult legal experts or your embassy for guidance on these laws. They can help you handle the details and ensure you make informed decisions.

BUILDING A SUPPORT NETWORK

1. **Find the Right Healthcare Provider**: To ensure clear communication and effective care, look for a healthcare provider who understands your needs and speaks your language.

2. **Join Local and Online Communities**: Connect with local expat groups and online communities for support and advice. These groups can offer invaluable insights and a sense of belonging.

3. **Create a Strong Support Network**: Build a network of friends, fellow expats, and local contacts to help you manage the challenges of living abroad. This support system will provide emotional and practical support.

By keeping these key points in mind, you can better prepare for maternity abroad. Hopefully, you already learned some useful information that can make your transition smoother and your experience more fulfilling in your new home.

PART 3
The Birthing Experience Abroad

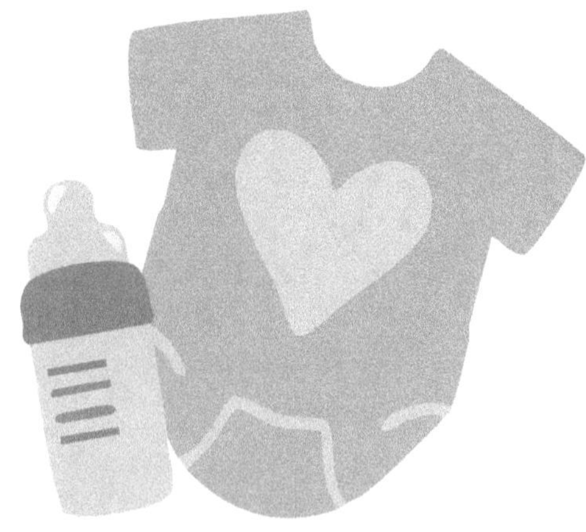

Every country has its own unique spin on childbirth. You won't only be dealing with different healthcare systems; you'll also be experiencing a blend of traditional and modern approaches that might be totally different from what you're used to.

Let's talk about all the **birthing options** you may come across in your new home. Whether you opt for a high-tech hospital, quaint birthing center, or the intimacy of a home birth, each setting offers its own set of perks and quirks. While making the correct choice may seem like a stressful task, this book is here to simplify the process by looking at these various options in detail. Plus, I've got some great stories from other foreign moms who have been right where you are. Their experiences could give you some invaluable insights into what to expect.

And then come the **cultural differences**—oh boy, they can really open your eyes! Some places lean toward very medical, by-the-book deliveries, while others might surprise you with more natural, community centered practices. Focus on finding a balance that feels right for you and adapting to the local customs.

How can you fully embrace this adventure, integrate some of your own traditions, and create a birth story that resonates with your new life abroad? Let's explore these ideas together. The goal here is to set you up to plan a birthing experience that's uniquely yours, even if you're miles away from home.

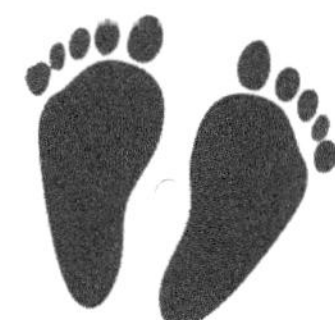

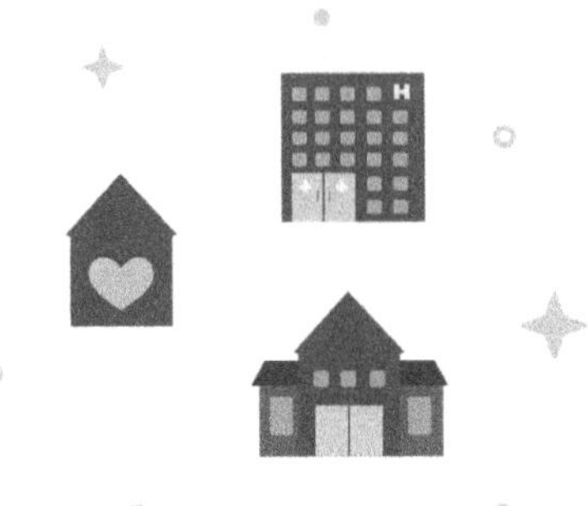

COMPARING BIRTHING OPTIONS: HOSPITALS, BIRTHING CENTERS, AND HOME BIRTHS

When you're gearing up for childbirth in a new country, one of the big choices you have to make is where to have your baby. That's a pretty significant decision, right? You've got hospitals, birthing centers, and even the option of a home birth. Each has its own vibe and set of benefits, and what you choose can depend on many different factors like medical recommendations, what makes you feel most comfortable, and even the local cultural norms. All these aspects may play a role in your decision-making process.

It's a lot to think about, so let me break it down for you. Where you decide to give birth isn't just about the place; it's also about setting the scene for your own experience and finding the right fit for you in this new setting.

Thankfully, expectant mothers can visit these places before making a decision. Getting a firsthand feel for these options before making your choice can help you feel more confident and comfortable with the process. Let's talk through the possibilities and find what feels best for you.

HOSPITALS

Hospitals can be a pretty solid choice for your big day, especially if you're the type who likes having all your bases covered. They're probably the best option for more complex pregnancies that need a bit more watching, or if you're thinking about pain relief options like epidurals.

Pros:

- You've got a full deck of medical services and emergency care right at your fingertips. It's basically your safety net.

- Pain relief options are plentiful, so if you're considering an epidural, you're all set in a hospital.

- This option is ideal for high-risk pregnancies, where having quick access to advanced care gives you peace of mind.

Cons:

- It might feel a bit clinical and impersonal. Hospitals are bustling places, and the atmosphere might not be as warm or personal as you'd like.

- The level of personalized care can be hit or miss. Depending on how busy the staff is, you might not get that cozy, one-on-one attention.

- There's often a higher chance of medical interventions being implemented, such as induced labor, epidurals, and cesarean sections, which might not always be necessary.

- Depending on your visa status, you might have to pay for these services out of pocket (true story).

In a hospital setting, you get the full medical experience with all the bells and whistles. Think of it as staying in a high-tech hotel with a lot of staff around. In the United States, for example, hospitals often have neonatal intensive care units (NICUs) ready for any newborns who may require extra care.

What to Expect:

- **Medical Staff**: You'll have obstetricians, nurses, anesthesiologists, and pediatricians on call in a hospital setting, so any unanticipated issues can be handled quickly.

- **Facilities**: Hospitals have high-tech equipment, operating rooms for C-sections, and plenty of pain relief options like epidurals.

- **Monitoring**: Expect continuous monitoring of your baby's heartbeat to catch any issues quickly.

- **Emergency Care**: You'll have instant access to emergency procedures if needed.

So, if you're leaning toward a hospital birth, it really boils down to what feels right for you and your baby.

Did you know that in the US, 98.4% of births happen in hospitals? However, that doesn't mean cesarean surgeries are taking over.[10] In fact, 68% of births were reported to be vaginal.[11] It's impossible to find out the reason behind these trends, since the choices mothers make are often influenced by doctors, insurers, and hospital rules. Advanced healthcare innovations like epidural anesthesia have made childbirth more controlled but also more clinical, pushing out midwifery and home births.

This trend isn't limited to the US. In Brazil, 55.7% of births are cesareans, the second-highest rate in the world. Low-income women in Brazil often rely on public hospitals that prefer vaginal births, while wealthier women in private hospitals choose cesareans as a status symbol.[12]

Danielle Rocha, who gave birth to her third child in South Africa in 2021, shared her experience: "In private hospitals, cesareans are common and often assumed unless you specifically request a natural birth. In public hospitals, most births are natural and typically without anesthesia." This was the opposite of her experience with her first two sons in the United States, where natural births were the norm, and cesareans were only performed when necessary. Her experience highlights the varying healthcare systems and birthing practices between the countries. In South Africa, 73% of private hospital births are cesareans, compared to 27.4% in public hospitals.[13]

Why are cesareans on the rise globally? Researchers are still figuring it out. It's not like they're automatically safer, as they come with risks like any major surgery. Some think it's because of fears about the risks of natural births. Others believe it's about mothers increasingly wanting more control over their delivery dates.[14] Flávia Imamura, a Brazilian mother in Japan, said there's a strong push for natural births there, but cesareans are more common than she expected. "The hospital where I gave birth has a rule: If your first child is born via cesarean, your next will be too. But they encourage natural births unless there are complications."

BIRTHING CENTERS

Birthing centers are like the cozy middle ground between a hospital and a home birth. They're perfect if you're aiming for a natural birth but still want some medical pros around just in case.

Pros:

- The vibe is more like being at home than in a medical facility, which can make the whole experience more relaxing.

- Birthing centers emphasize natural birthing methods, so if you're looking to go medication-free, this could be your spot.

Cons:

- These are not the best option for high-risk pregnancies. If you or the baby might need extra medical attention during or after delivery, a birthing center might not have facilities that match the level of a hospital.

- Pain relief options are more limited. If you think you might want an epidural, for example, you won't find that here.

- In case of complications, you might need to be transferred to a hospital, which can add stress during what's already a pretty intense time.

- Birthing centers can be either paid or covered by insurance, depending on your plan and location. It's important to check the costs involved and whether your insurance will cover them.

Birthing centers in places like Canada offer a cozy, home-like atmosphere with professional care, focusing on a natural birthing process in a relaxed environment. Sounds lovely, right? But, heads up—birthing centers aren't as common everywhere else as they are in Canada. Cultural norms and regulations around childbirth can vary, so these centers might not always be an option.

For instance, in some places, hospital births are the go-to. Take Italy, for example. About 98% of births happen in hospitals there.[15] Although the number of birthing centers in Italy has gradually increased in recent years, they are still quite rare compared to other countries.

So, what's a soon-to-be parent to do? This is where your detective skills come in handy. When you're planning to give birth abroad, a little personal research goes a long way. Check out local healthcare options, chat with healthcare providers, and join expat parent groups. You might even want to visit potential birthing spots to see what feels right for you. With a bit of legwork, you can find the best fit for your birthing experience, no matter which country you find yourself in.

What to Expect:

- **Medical Staff**: Certified nurse-midwives or midwives will oversee your birth experience, sometimes with obstetricians on call.

- **Facilities**: Birthing centers have comfy rooms with options for water births, birthing balls, and other natural comfort measures.

- **Monitoring**: Expect intermittent monitoring, which means more freedom to move.

- **Emergency Protocols**: Have plans in place for quick transfer to a hospital if needed.

Birthing centers offer a sweet spot, as they allow you to take a natural approach, while always accounting for safety. They're all about that comfy atmosphere with a touch of medical backup when you need it. What do you think? Does the more homely feel appeal to you, or does the idea of potential transfers make you nervous?

Did you know the annual number of births recorded in birth centers in the United States grew by 65% from 2011 to 2021?[16] Giving birth in a comfortable, home-like atmosphere is becoming increasingly popular in Switzerland too. In 2016, 1,769 babies were born in these centers, making up about 70% of all non-clinical deliveries and almost 2% of total deliveries in Switzerland.[17]

Flávia Imamura summed up her experience with the medical facilities available in Japan perfectly: "Here in Okinawa, there's a very famous clinic that's really sought after, especially by foreigners. It has a very natural, cozy atmosphere, like a little Japanese traditional wooden house, but it's a fully-equipped medical facility." I don't know about you, but I find something about the Japanese aesthetic very serene.

HOME BIRTHS

Oh, home births! They offer a cozy, intimate environment where you can bring new life into the world. Having your baby at home can be perfect if you've had a low-risk pregnancy and are expecting a similar delivery. The focus is on creating a personal and comfortable experience, where you control the atmosphere from start to finish.

Pros:

- You're in your own space, which can make the whole experience feel more intimate and less stressful.

- You get ultra-personalized care directly from a midwife or a qualified birth attendant who's there just for you.

- It puts you in the driver's seat for your birthing process. You decide what happens and when, without the usual hospital protocols.

Cons:

- It's best for pregnancies without complications. If things get tricky, you'd need to switch gears quickly.

- If you need medical intervention suddenly, the process of receiving care may not be as swift as it would be in a hospital.

- Depending on where you are in the world, people might have mixed feelings about home births. In some places, it's quite common; in others, not so much.

- Hiring a midwife, doula, or nurse to assist with a home birth can be an added expense. Be sure to check whether your insurance covers this cost.

In the UK, home births are popular for low-risk pregnancies and are supported by midwives who bring all the necessary supplies to your home.

What to Expect:

- **Medical Staff**: Midwives or trained birth attendants come to your home.

- **Facilities**: You give birth in your own home, with options like rented birthing pools and other comfort items.

- **Monitoring**: Expect intermittent monitoring, similar to birthing centers.

- **Emergency Protocols**: Have a solid plan for hospital transfer if needed.

Did you know in the Netherlands, home birth (*thuisbevalling* in Dutch) is quite popular, with about 30% of women choosing to deliver at home?[18] This statistic doesn't only reflect tradition; it reflects a broader philosophy that sees childbirth as a natural, family-centered event rather than a medical procedure.

In fact, this philosophy is deeply ingrained in Dutch society and is backed by a strong primary care system. The Dutch midwifery model, which oversees home births, emphasizes minimal intervention and lets mothers give birth in a familiar, comfortable environment. They really trust the natural birthing process and have a great support network for both prenatal and postnatal care.

Deciding where to give birth is entirely personal, right? You've got to make your decision based on your comfort, your health, the risks, and what's available around you. It's always a good idea to chat with your healthcare provider to figure out the best plan for you. So, at this point, what feels right to you?

Cultural Differences in Birthing Practices: How to Advocate for Your Birthing Plan

Cultural norms and practices surrounding childbirth can affect every aspect of the birthing process, from the role of the partner during labor to the use of pain relief interventions and the practices immediately following birth. Understanding these differences is an important part of preparing for your birthing experience abroad and making sure you don't encounter any hiccups.

Advocating for your birthing plan in a foreign healthcare system requires clear communication and at times negotiation. You must:

- **Educate yourself** about the local birthing practices and healthcare system.

- **Communicate your preferences** clearly with your healthcare provider. Consider hiring a translator if you encounter a language barrier.

- **Be flexible**, understanding that some aspects of your plan may need to adapt to the local context.

- **Seek support** from local expat groups, who can offer advice and share their experiences.

NAVIGATING PAIN MANAGEMENT OPTIONS

Pain management during labor is a highly personal choice and can be influenced by cultural norms, personal preferences, and medical necessity. Options may include:

- **Breathing Techniques:** Controlled breathing patterns such as slow, deep breaths or quick, shallow breaths can help manage pain and promote relaxation during labor.[20]
  - **Pros:** Encourages the baby's descent, can reduce the need for medical interventions, and promotes a sense of control.

  - **Cons:** May not provide sufficient pain relief for some women, and requires training, practice, and concentration.

- **Movement:** Changing positions, walking, swaying, or rocking can help ease discomfort and facilitate labor progress.[21]
  - **Pros:** Encourages the baby's descent, can reduce the need for medical interventions, and promotes a sense of control.

  - **Cons:** May become tiring. Some positions may not be possible with certain medical conditions or interventions, and the results of this technique can depend on the person's pain tolerance. Depending on the setting, some positions may not be allowed or feasible.

- **Hydrotherapy:** Laboring in a warm bath or shower can provide relaxation and pain relief and promote labor progress.[22]

- **Pros:** Non-pharmacological and can reduce the need for medical interventions. This technique promotes relaxation and comfort.

- **Cons:** Not available in all birth settings. May require assistance to ensure safety, and water temperature must be carefully regulated.

- **Epidurals:** A regional anesthesia injected into the area around the spinal cord, providing numbness from the waist down.[23]
  - **Pros:** Highly effective pain relief. This option allows the mother to rest and conserve energy, and the strength can be adjusted depending on her pain tolerance.

  - **Cons:** May slow labor progress and cause temporary side effects like itching or shivering. Requires continuous monitoring.

- **Spinal Blocks:** A single shot of anesthesia injected directly into the spinal fluid provides rapid pain relief, although for a shorter duration than an epidural.[24]
  - **Pros:** Fast-acting, can be used for instrumental or cesarean deliveries, and allows the mother to be awake and alert.

  - **Cons:** Cannot be easily adjusted or extended, may cause temporary side effects like itching or nausea, and requires careful timing of administration.

- **Nitrous Oxide:** A gas mixture of nitrous oxide and oxygen, inhaled through a mask to provide short-term pain relief.[25]
  - **Pros:** Can be self-administered, takes effect quickly, and does not interfere with labor progress or mobility.

  - **Cons:** May cause dizziness or nausea, does not provide complete pain relief, and is not available in all birth settings.

Don't wait until it's time to deliver. Instead, get on top of things by starting a conversation with your healthcare provider today about your pain management options, including natural birthing methods and the possibility of a cesarean section. Understanding what's available to you can help you create a birthing experience that aligns with your wishes and needs.

THE ROLE OF PARTNERS AND SUPPORT PERSONS

Partners' and support persons' level of involvement during labor and delivery can differ widely across cultures. In some places, partners are expected to be deeply involved; they attend prenatal classes and offer hands-on support throughout labor. However, in other cultures, the partner's role might be less active, or they might even be excluded from the birthing room entirely.

To avoid any confusion, talk to your healthcare provider and the birthing facility well in advance to clarify the expectations and policies concerning the presence of partners and support persons. If it's important to you that your partner or a chosen support person—such as a parent or friend—is present, you may have to advocate for your needs. This is one of the reasons why it is important to get these details sorted well ahead of time.

Cintia, living in Portugal, recounts her experience: "As I paced back and forth across the room during contractions, I was grateful to be in the last room, giving us plenty of space to move. My husband was right there with me, matching my steps and supporting me through each contraction. Together, we moved rhythmically, side by side, which made the intense moments more bearable." This is just one of the many examples of how the labor process can become easier with an active partner's support.

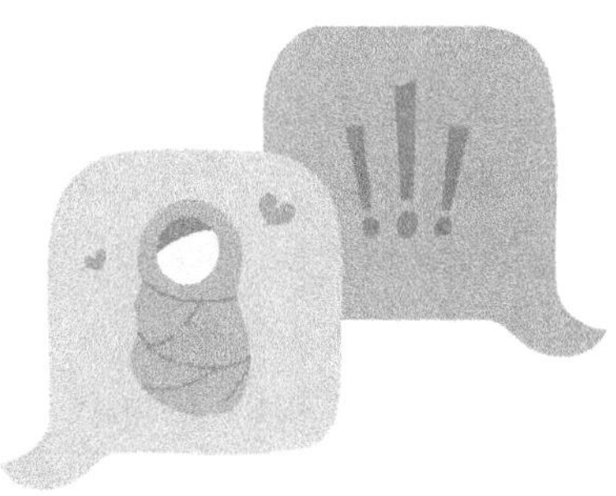

Childbirth in the Land of Windmills: A Real-life tale

If you had seen Cauê squeezing all those bags, pillows, blankets, and a giant ball into the trunk of his car, you might have guessed he was packing for a fun week at the beach, but that wasn't the case.

His wife Alana, who was 39 weeks pregnant, watched him go back and forth from their house, meticulously checking off items from her 'better be prepared than sorry' maternity list. "Don't forget the inflatable pool," she reminded him with a wave of her finger, determined to make sure nothing went wrong.

Alana wanted to be in a place that felt like home with all its comforts. She did a lot of research and mapped out possible restaurants around the hospital, in case food delivery wasn't an option. The hospital had cafeterias, but she wanted backup plans just in case. She wanted to have the perfect experience. So, it made sense that the list was long. Although getting everything under control was exhausting, the peace of mind was worth it. Squeezing her favorite pillow between her arms, she hopped into the car, and off they went to the hospital to start the induction.

The truth was Alana didn't initially like the idea of a Foley's balloon induction. "I always thought about natural birth with less medical intervention," she recalls. A Foley's balloon induction involves inserting a small balloon catheter into the cervix and inflating it to help the cervix dilate[19]. Basically, it's a mechanical method used to induce labor without medication. "It's a mechanical thing; it's not medicine, but it's a mechanical intervention happening to your body."

But the induction wasn't something she was obligated to accept. "I remember calling a number ... I don't know how to explain what it is, but it's a number for volunteers who are midwives and gynecologists. And I'm very much about numbers and data to make decisions. So, I called this number and talked to someone. When I spoke with this person—a completely random person who wasn't biased in any way, you know?—I felt more confident with the process. So, I went to the hospital and said, 'I want the induction.' I packed my entire house, even my birthing tub, which I had rented. I said, "I'm going to the hospital with everything." And she really did.

At the hospital, she laid down with her legs wide open and in the air. You know what I'm talking about—that position any shy or reserved person would never want to assume in front of two unknown nurses. But there was Alana, getting ready for the Foley balloon. Although Alana did her due research before the procedure, she found it to be more challenging than expected. She had read that it wouldn't hurt, but the reality was different. Holding her husband's hand, she whispered, "It's painful!"

"You need to relax a little," said the nurse standing in front of her. At that moment, Alana felt a warm wave of positive energy envelop her, as if her body was telling her to "embrace it."

"It wasn't the birth of my dreams, but it was the birth that was meant to be. The important thing was that I would see my baby soon," Alana reflected. And she was right. In less than two hours, she began to have contractions, which was a lot quicker than the doctors expected—they believed things wouldn't progress until the next day.

Using guided meditation, she calmed herself and managed to sleep, only to wake up when her water broke. "I told my husband, 'If I ask for anesthesia three times, at least twenty minutes apart each time, then call someone.' I really wanted to experience everything fully. I had a doula, which I highly recommend. She was my angel. She knew my birth plan; it was amazing."

"When I was five centimeters dilated, the midwife suggested we set up the bathtub. I stayed in the bathtub until I was exhausted. My midwife then suggested trying the bed. Three minutes after moving to the bed, my baby was born."

Alana's story shows how careful planning, flexibility, and support make the birthing experience abroad easier and better. Whether in a hospital, birthing center, or at home, understanding the local approach and preparing for various scenarios can lead to a birth that feels right for you and your baby.

Something to Keep in Mind

Parents should also have a backup plan in case something goes wrong during labor. No matter where or how you decide to have the baby, consider the following:

- **Know the Nearest Hospital**: Even if you plan a home birth or a birthing center delivery, know the quickest route to the nearest hospital in case of an emergency.

- **Emergency Contacts**: Keep a list of emergency contacts ready, including numbers for your healthcare provider, midwife, and a close family member or friend who can be there to support you.

- **Birth Plan Flexibility**: While having a birth plan is great, stay flexible and open to medical interventions if they become necessary for the safety of you or your baby.

- **Transport Arrangements**: Ensure you have reliable transportation available at all times. Consider arranging for a trusted friend or family member to drive you if possible—app drivers can sometimes get lost on their way to the hospital (true story from a friend of mine). And whatever you do, please don't consider driving yourself! Cintia, in Portugal, once told me that on the day she went into labor, she felt perfectly fine between contractions and insisted she could drive herself to the hospital. Thankfully, she came to her senses for the sake of everyone on the road and inside the car!

- **Essential Items**: Have a hospital bag packed with essentials, even if you plan to give birth at home or a birthing center.

By considering these factors and being prepared for any situation, you can help ensure a smoother and safer birthing experience.

Summary of Key Points

UNDERSTANDING YOUR BIRTHING OPTIONS

Hospitals

- **Pros**: It's a five-star hotel with all the amenities—pain relief, emergency care, and lots of staff to cater to you.

- **Cons**: It can feel a bit like a busy airport terminal with lots of people and noise. It's not always super cozy.

Birthing Centers

- **Pros**: Think of it as cozy, homey, and perfect for a natural birth with some medical backup.

- **Cons**: If complications arise, you might need to shift to a hospital, which can be stressful.

Home Births

- **Pros**: Ultimate comfort—your home, your rules.

- **Cons**: Great for low-risk pregnancies, but if complications arise, you'll need to quickly get to the hospital, which can be stressful.

EMBRACING CULTURAL DIFFERENCES AND ADVOCATING FOR YOUR BIRTH PLAN

- **Understand Local Practices**: Get to know the local customs and protocols to understand how things work so you can fit in smoothly.

- **Clear Communication**: Speak up about your needs and preferences. Make sure you're clear and precise about what you want.

- **Seek Support**: Join local expatriate groups to find a community of people who understand your situation and can offer support.

NAVIGATING PAIN MANAGEMENT OPTIONS

- **Non-Pharmacological**: Breathing techniques, movement, and hydrotherapy

- **Pharmacological**: Epidurals, spinal blocks, and nitrous oxide

THE ROLE OF PARTNERS AND SUPPORT PERSONS

- **Partner Involvement**: Make sure your partner knows they're on duty. Their support is crucial during this time.

- **Active Support**: Your partner can be your biggest cheerleader and support system, providing encouragement and help whenever you need it.

By keeping these points in mind, you'll be ready to handle the birthing experience abroad. Think of it as planning a big trip. Once everything is set, it's smooth sailing (or as smooth as childbirth can be)!

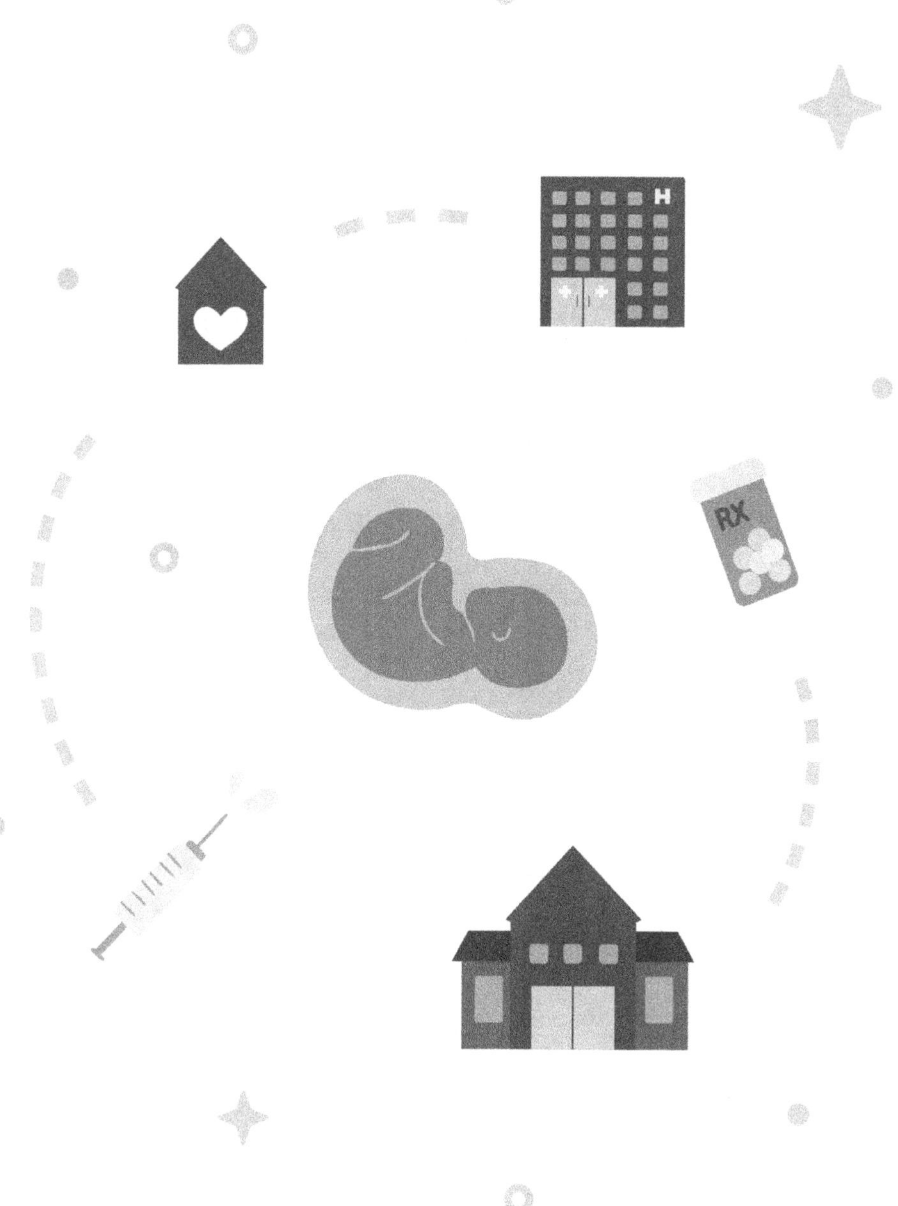

PART 4
Postpartum support and practices

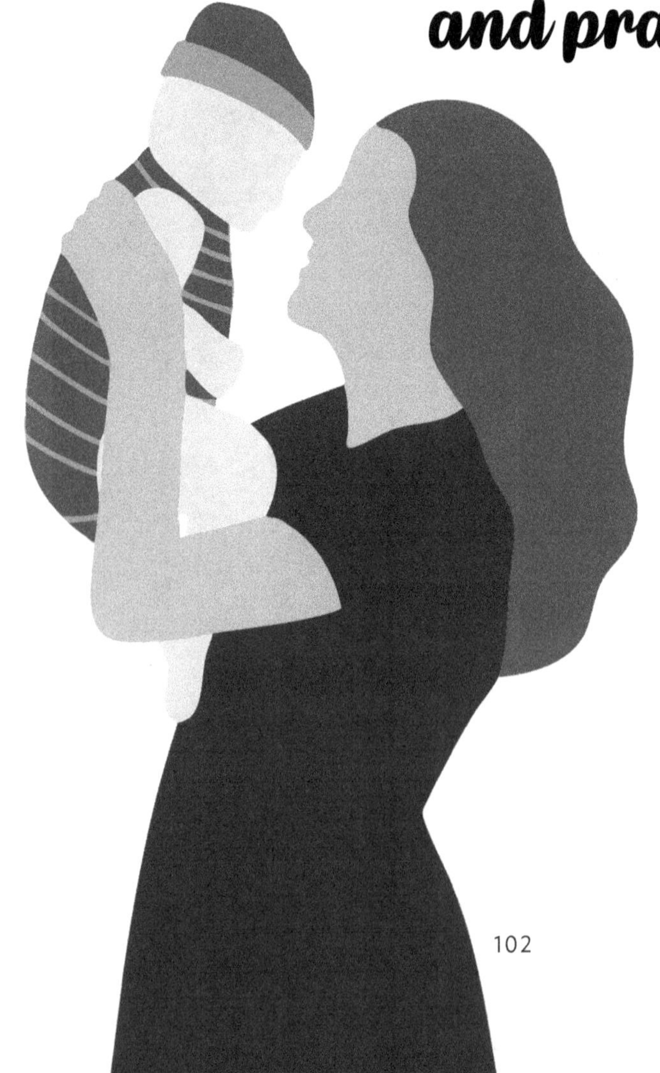

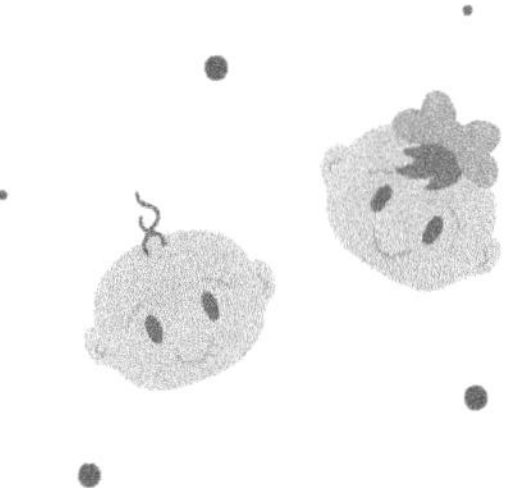

The period following childbirth, often referred to as the postpartum period, is a time of considerable physical and emotional adjustment for new mothers. Across the globe, cultures have developed unique practices and traditions to support women during this challenging time. Experiencing postpartum care in a foreign country presents both challenges and opportunities. By blending traditional wisdom with modern healthcare practices, you can make the most of your resources. Let's look at a few important topics such as the essentials of **postpartum care,** diverse cultural practices, and creating a **supportive community** abroad.

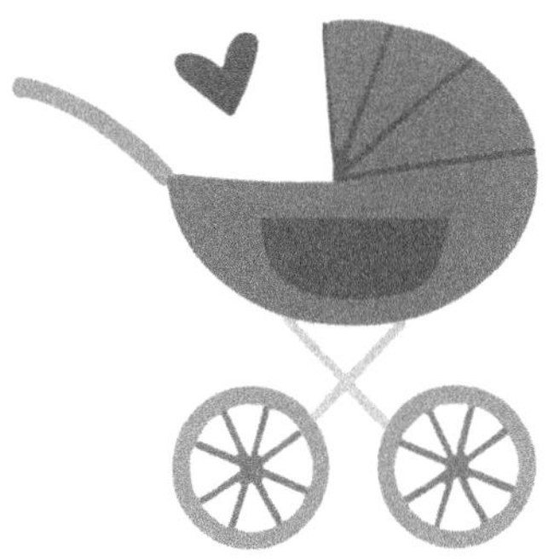

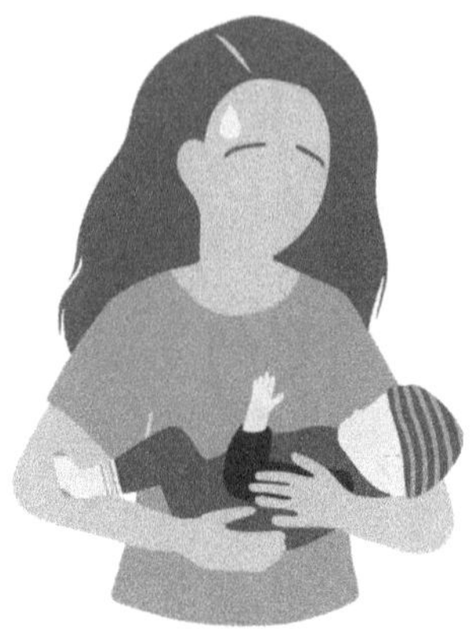

POSTPARTUM CARE FOR MOTHERS:

The postpartum period requires attentive care for the mother's physical recovery, even as she adjusts to motherhood on an emotional level. Access to and the quality of postpartum care can vary greatly from country to country, and understanding the local healthcare system is necessary to get through this period successfully. Two types of resources are necessary to make this stage less stressful: physical health resources and mental health support.

Physical health resources might include postnatal checkups, rehabilitation services for pelvic floor recovery, and lactation consultants for breastfeeding support. Many countries offer home visits by midwives or nurses in the first weeks after birth, providing important support and monitoring for both mother and baby.

Mental health support is equally important, as many new mothers may experience the "baby blues," and some may even develop postpartum depression or anxiety. Familiarizing yourself with the available mental health services, including counseling and support groups, is a vital step in preparing for the postpartum period. Mothers living in a foreign country should request access to professionals who can speak their language if needed and explore online resources and communities for broader support options.

UNDERSTANDING AND ADAPTING TO LOCAL POSTPARTUM PRACTICES

A look at the postpartum practices around the world can be quite interesting, since it provides information about the different cultural values related to motherhood and child-rearing. In addition to supporting new mothers, these customs also reflect each community's lifestyle and beliefs.

For instance, Latin American countries observe the *cuarentena*, a restorative 40-day period post-birth where mothers rest and bond with their babies. In contrast, some Asian cultures focus on the mother's recovery through a strict confinement period, which involves special diets and rituals. These customs show how community plays an important role in shaping the postpartum experience.

The Netherlands also has an interesting custom in place—the *Kraamzorg* system—to support new mothers. In this practice, a trained nurse assists the new mother for eight to ten days after birth. This nurse offers guidance and support with everything from infant care to household tasks. Alana appreciated the practical support soon after her hospital discharge, noting, "My *Kraamzorg* showed me how to change a diaper and bathe my son, and more importantly, she supported me as a mother."

TIPS FOR NAVIGATING LOCAL POSTPARTUM PRACTICES:

- **Research Beforehand:** Understand your host country's postpartum customs to make sure your expectations are accurate. Doing so will help you prepare adequately.

- **Find Local Support Networks:** Connect with local maternal figures, postpartum doulas, or community groups who respect your cultural preferences to make sure the support you receive is more personalized.

- **Communicate Openly:** Discuss your comfort levels and expectations with healthcare providers to personalize your postpartum care.

- **Blend Customs with Personal Beliefs:** Embracing local customs is always fun. However, to make your postpartum journey less stressful, adapt them in ways that align with your own cultural and personal beliefs. Always look for support groups that make you feel comfortable and supported. Keep in mind that some online communities can be judgmental or combative, so focus on finding a group that builds positivity and trust. Avoid absorbing too much negativity, and remember that your approach to parenting should feel right for you and your family.

- **Seek Professional Guidance:** When trying to figure out both legal and medical rights, it's natural to feel overwhelmed. Try reaching out for professional advice or contacting your embassy for help.

By blending local customs with personal preferences, non-native mothers can ensure a recovery that is both culturally respectful and personally satisfying. Whether you decide to stick to local traditions or modify them to fit your personal needs, the goal is a postpartum experience that supports both mother and child in the best possible way.

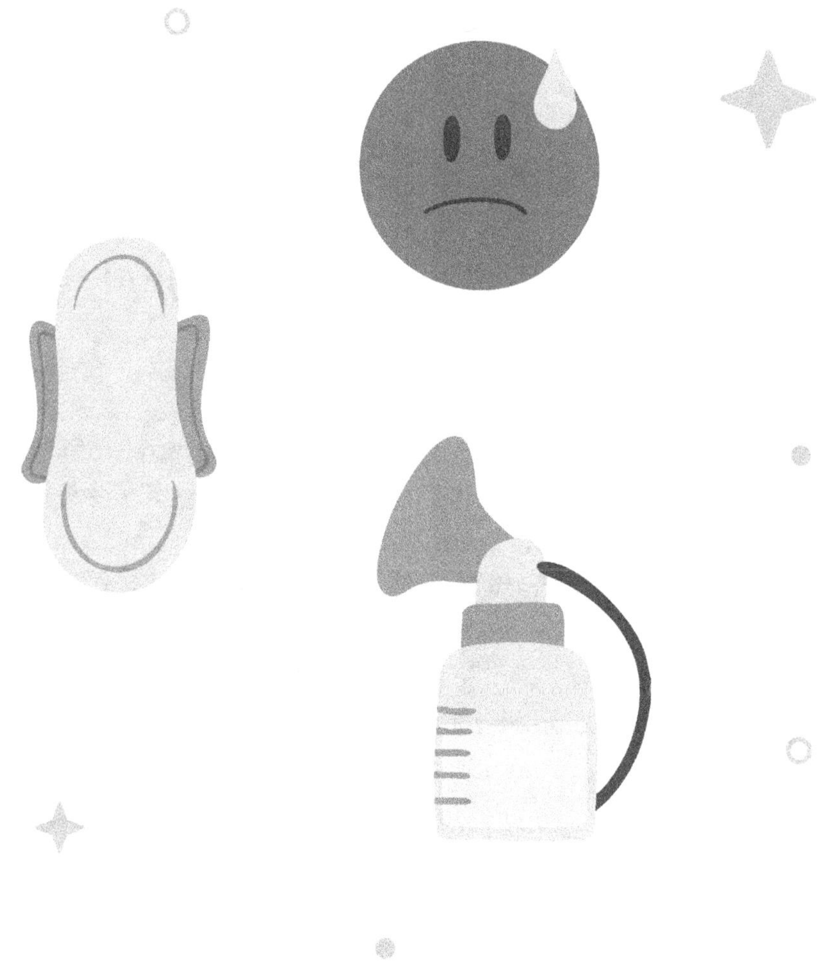

BALANCING INTERCULTURAL FAMILY DYNAMICS

At this stage of our journey, we have another central topic to explore: how intercultural couples and families often have different notions and expectations regarding traditions and practices. Take Ana Flavia, for example. She's from Brazil, her husband is from India, and they live in the United States. Ana shared, "Our approach to pregnancy and the first year of a baby's life differs significantly from the cultures I come from and live in." It was not uncommon for the couple to have discussions about what each culture expects and how those expectations fit with their family values. Success looks like finding that sweet spot of compromise and making sure everyone feels respected.

CULTURAL EXPECTATIONS AND COMPROMISE

For example, in Indian culture, it's customary to shave a one-year-old's head as part of a traditional ceremony. Ana mentioned, "For me, this practice feels too drastic and invasive, so I have already decided that we won't be shaving our baby's hair." It's very important to engage in these discussions early on, so both partners feel respected and heard.

EXTENDED FAMILY INVOLVEMENT

Not only the couple needs to discuss these traditions—more often than not, negotiations will involve grandparents and extended family members as well. Different generations can have strong views on cultural practices, so managing these expectations requires sensitivity and diplomacy.

TIPS FOR INTERCULTURAL NEGOTIATIONS

- **Open Communication**: Ensure both partners share their cultural expectations and boundaries openly and honestly.

- **Educate Each Other**: Take the time to learn about each other's cultural practices to understand the significance behind them.

- **Seek Compromise**: Work together to find a middle ground where both cultural practices can be respected or combined.

- **Set Boundaries**: Agree on non-negotiables to avoid future conflicts and misunderstandings.

- **Involve Extended Family**: Have open discussions with extended family to manage their expectations and explain your joint decisions.

While intercultural families face unique challenges, they can be handled smoothly if you work as a team. When you do so, you're working toward a more harmonious family environment that can enrich your experience living abroad.

CREATING A SENSE OF COMMUNITY: FINDING AND OFFERING SUPPORT TO OTHER INTERNATIONAL MOTHERS

The postpartum period can be isolating, especially for non-natives who are far from their usual support networks. Thankfully, you can create a new support network where you are, even as you navigate life and parenthood so far away from home. Establishing or joining a community with other mothers who are also finding their place on foreign soil can provide invaluable support during this vulnerable time. Such communities go a long way in creating safe spaces where you can share experiences, exchange advice, and form meaningful connections.

FINDING YOUR COMMUNITY

You can start building your support network with simple online searches for local expat parent groups, which are often abundant and welcoming. Social media platforms and foreign-focused websites are excellent resources. Expatriate groups are particularly valuable because they understand the unique challenges you're facing.

You can also meet other expectant mothers going through similar life changes by attending prenatal classes. Another obvious benefit of this resource is that it prepares you for childbirth. Additionally, joining local clubs or participating in family-oriented activities can help you and your family integrate into the community and make lasting friendships.

GIVING SUPPORT TO OTHERS

Offering support to fellow expatriates helps them deal with hurdles you may have encountered before. At the same time, it's a great way to enhance your sense of belonging and purpose. Sharing your experiences, providing a listening ear, or helping newcomers figure out the local healthcare system are all ways to forge strong connections. Both you and the newcomers can benefit from this mutually supportive relationship.

By actively engaging in or starting such groups, you contribute to building a welcoming space that brings with it the familiar comforts of home. These networks transform the challenging task of handling maternity abroad into a collective effort filled with empathy and companionship.

Remember, every act of kindness, no matter how small, can significantly impact those adapting to motherhood away from their home country. Through these networks, foreign mothers find not just practical help but also hope and a sense of extended family, which are essential for thriving in a new environment.

Supporting You – the New Mom

Let's be real for a second here. If you don't tell people what you need, you might end up with a giant plush unicorn, which may be cute, but isn't exactly useful when you're trying to manage a newborn! While being direct about your needs can be difficult sometimes, it's important to make this scary stage a little less stressful. Still skeptical? Just ask my friend Debora—she'll tell you all about the giant plush unicorn I gave her, when she really could have used diapers and baby wipes instead! So, don't be shy when someone asks how they can help. Or better yet, pass this book to your friend, family member (if they're coming to stay with you), or even a work colleague (why not, right?) and I'll let them know how to support you.

- **Emotional Support**: Catching the curveballs pregnancy throws can be challenging enough without the added burden of living far away from home. Luckily, you can find ways to receive emotional support from your loved ones despite the miles of distance. If you need someone to talk to, just grab your phone and ask. While it may feel awkward at first, it will make you feel much better in the long run.

- **Household Help**

  - **Cooking and Meals**: If you've been living in your neighborhood for a while, you likely have a good community already that is likely to offer help after the delivery. Usually, that help comes in the form of good, home-cooked meals. Accept such gestures with gratitude, as it eliminates the stress of cooking. If you've just moved to a new country and don't know a lot of people there, discuss the option of ordering in meals with your partner. If your family wants to do something nice from back home, consider asking them to have your breakfast delivered using food delivery apps. I received one on my first day back from the hospital, and it was everything. It felt like a warm hug, and the note from my friend was the positive assurance I needed.

- **Cleaning**: Managing household chores like cleaning, laundry, and grocery shopping can get very tricky once the baby arrives. This is a good time to ask your partner or your close friends to step in and get some of these tasks off the to-do list. If that's not an option, create a mom support registry for those who want to send in gifts to celebrate your new bundle of joy.

  The list can include items that will make your life easier, like a robot vacuum cleaner. Believe me; my robot vacuum is still my hero to this day.

- **Running Errands**: Running errands with a newborn isn't an option, right? Your partner or your neighbors can take that off your plate too. You just need to ask. Maybe your neighbor is heading to the farmer's market today; if so, ask him or her to grab a few healthy veggies for you.

- **Baby Care**
  - **Holding the Baby**: As a new mom, being separated from the baby, even for a couple of minutes, can be stressful. But when guests offer to hold your baby, I say jump at that opportunity to rest or take a shower. Your mind and body will thank you later.

  - **Night Shifts**: As I said before, you can forget getting a night of uninterrupted sleep after the baby arrives. So, if a friend or a family member decides to visit, take the opportunity to relax for one night by asking for their help and support. If you choose to breastfeed, maybe help with diaper changes or rocking the baby back to sleep during the night can help too.

- **Health and Well-Being**

  - **Encourage Self-Care:** Every mom needs some alone time, even if it's just for a short walk or a quiet cup of tea. When people you trust visit you, ask them to keep an eye on your baby, so you can take a few minutes for self-care.

  - **Appointments:** Medical appointments with a newborn can be anxiety-provoking and chaotic. An extra hand can make things easier and help you declutter your mind to a certain extent. Ask your work bestie or that kind elderly neighbor to accompany you.

- **Practical Advice and Information:**

  - **Local Resources:** Get in touch with other moms you know (or through online forums) to ask for info about local parenting groups, healthcare services, and baby-friendly places.

  - **Cultural Adaptation:** If you need help working through any cultural differences in parenting practices and healthcare, speak to your local friends. They can help you make sense of it all.

- **Supporting Siblings:** Finally, if you already have other kid(s), making sure their needs are met while you take care of your newborn can be difficult. Once in a while, you can ask your friends to take them out for activities or help with their routines. Arrange playdates with their friends (not at your house, if possible), so you get some time to focus solely on the baby.

- **Flexibility and Patience:** Your needs may change daily, so please ask your loved ones to be adaptable during this stage.

By offering this kind of support, friends and family can help new mothers feel less isolated and more capable of handling the challenges of new motherhood in a foreign country.

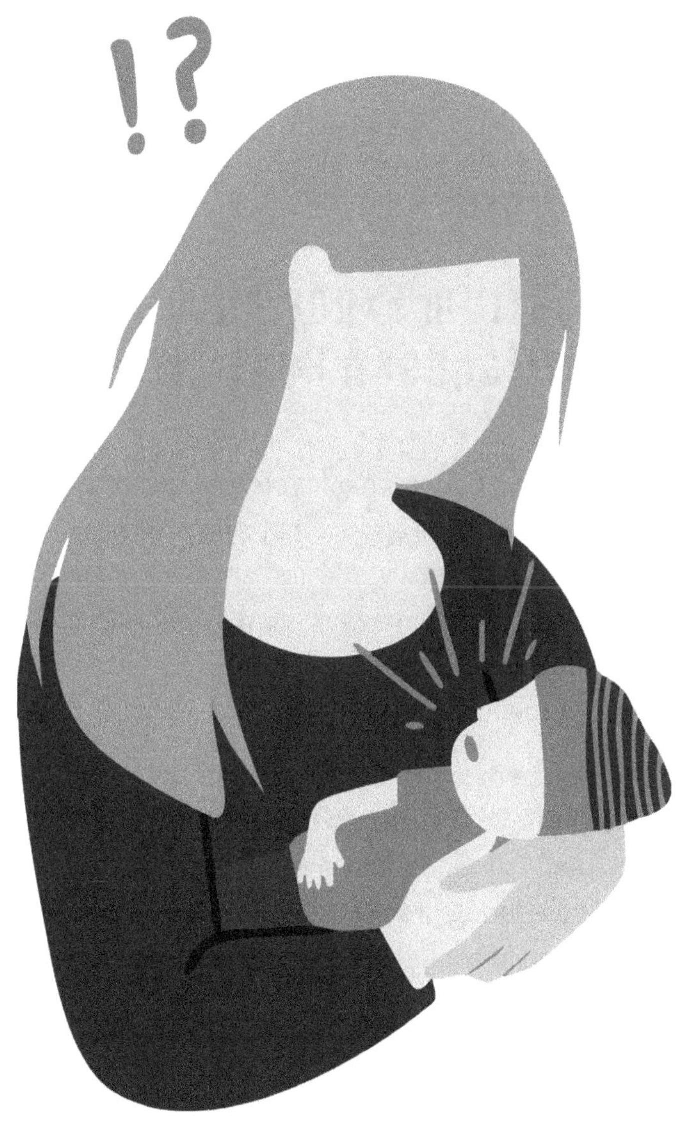

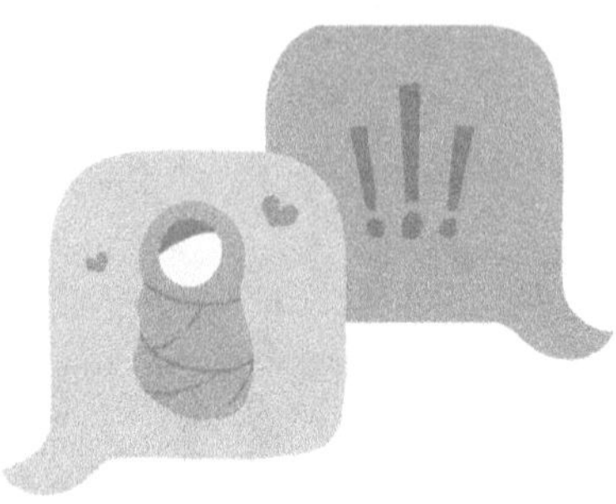

Postpartum Experience in the Netherlands: A Real-Life Tale

"Dear Rana, Bruno, and Olivia, thank you for your hospitality and for entrusting the care of your baby to a maternity nurse in training. Your home was a wonderful place to work. You are a warm family. I wish you much love, health, and happiness with your sweet Olivia." Anette read aloud, her Dutch accent lending a comforting rhythm to the words despite a few mispronunciations.

Rana, recording the moment on her phone, felt a wave of exhaustion mixed with contentment. The past two weeks had been a whirlwind of new experiences and emotions, and Anette, the family's *kraamzorg*, had been a constant, reassuring presence. Now, Anette stood before them, holding a handwritten letter.

As Anette's words filled the room, Rana felt a lump in her throat. She hadn't expected this level of warmth and gratitude. Tears welled up in her eyes; she was overwhelmed by a profound sense of connection and appreciation for Anette's care.

Rana had never imagined that a caregiver from another culture could have such a profound impact on her. Back in Brazil, her home country, such services would typically be handled by family members, or, if the family could afford them, a babysitter or cleaning person. Even then, it wouldn't have been the same. "I didn't have many expectations," Rana admitted, recalling her initial skepticism. "I had heard good things, but also vague reassurances like, 'Oh, it will help you.' I wasn't expecting such an excellent experience. I had my reservations about how Olivia should be cared for—things I didn't want done and things I wanted done. I was a bit defensive."

But now Annette was standing in her living room, bidding farewell with heartfelt words. It was safe to say that Anette's gentle demeanor had melted away those early reservations. Rana looked at Bruno, her husband, whose eyes reflected their shared gratitude and relief.

Anette, who had spent years in the Dutch flower industry before changing careers, had been under supervision during her time with Rana, Olivia, and Bruno, yet her presence had been invaluable. Rana's mother and younger sister were also there, sharing this emotional moment.

The family had been ready to support Rana and Olivia, but Anette had made a significant difference. On the day they were sent home from the hospital, Anette had arrived about an hour later to help. Rana had some experience with babies, since she had helped out her cousins before, but she admitted it wasn't enough, especially not at this level. It had been a cold day in the Netherlands when they brought the baby home, and not knowing much, they had left newborn Olivia in front of an open window. Luckily, Anette had arrived in time to prevent Olivia's temperature from dropping. She had helped with the baby and ensured Rana got some rest during those first days, even though Rana had tried to resist. "I should've rested more. I was always up, trying to do things," she admitted.

"She also saved my breastfeeding experience," confessed Rana. After thirty-six hours of labor at the hospital, Rana had struggled with breastfeeding due to an improper latch. But Anette had been determined to help, and thankfully, everything had improved from there. Well ... except for Olivia's soccer uniform, which her father had bought for her to wear for his favorite soccer team. That had a little incident which might have left a stain or two.

Rana's experience with Anette highlighted how embracing local postpartum practices, like the *Kraamzorg* system, can make a big difference in postpartum care as a means of providing both practical support and emotional comfort.

Summary of Key Points

UNDERSTANDING HEALTHCARE SYSTEMS AND POSTPARTUM CARE

Physical Health Resources

- **Postpartum Care:** Postnatal checkups, pelvic floor rehab, and lactation consultants are an important part of your recovery. They're available to help you heal and keep you feeling your best.

Mental Health Support

- Don't let the baby blues get you down. Scope out counseling and support groups like you're hunting for the best brunch spot. Remember, mental health is just as important as physical health!

NAVIGATING POSTPARTUM PRACTICES

Cultural Insights

- **Embrace Local Customs:** Explore local customs and traditions. The *cuarentena* in Latin America or the Dutch *Kraamzorg* might seem unfamiliar, but they're full of wisdom. Embrace the experience!

Adapt and Blend

- **Create New Traditions:** Mix and match local traditions with your own. If you don't have a lot of your own traditions, that's okay—you can create new ones! Combining local customs with new ideas can lead to unique and meaningful family traditions that fit your new life perfectly. Reaching out to friends and family for their suggestions can also help you build these new traditions.

Find Local Networks:

- **Join Mom Clubs and Community Groups:** It's like finding your own support squad, buzzing with baby talk instead of game strategies.

Building a Support Network

- **Find Your Tribe**: Join local expat parent groups, attend prenatal classes, and dive into community activities to build your own "mom squad"—stronger together!

- **Offer Support**: Share your experiences and help other newcomers. Be the wise elder of the tribe, guiding the newbies with your sage advice and hilarious anecdotes.

By keeping these key points in mind, you'll be well-prepared to get through the postpartum period in a foreign country. Think of it as an adventure in the postpartum playground—full of new friends, fun challenges, and plenty of laughs along the way.

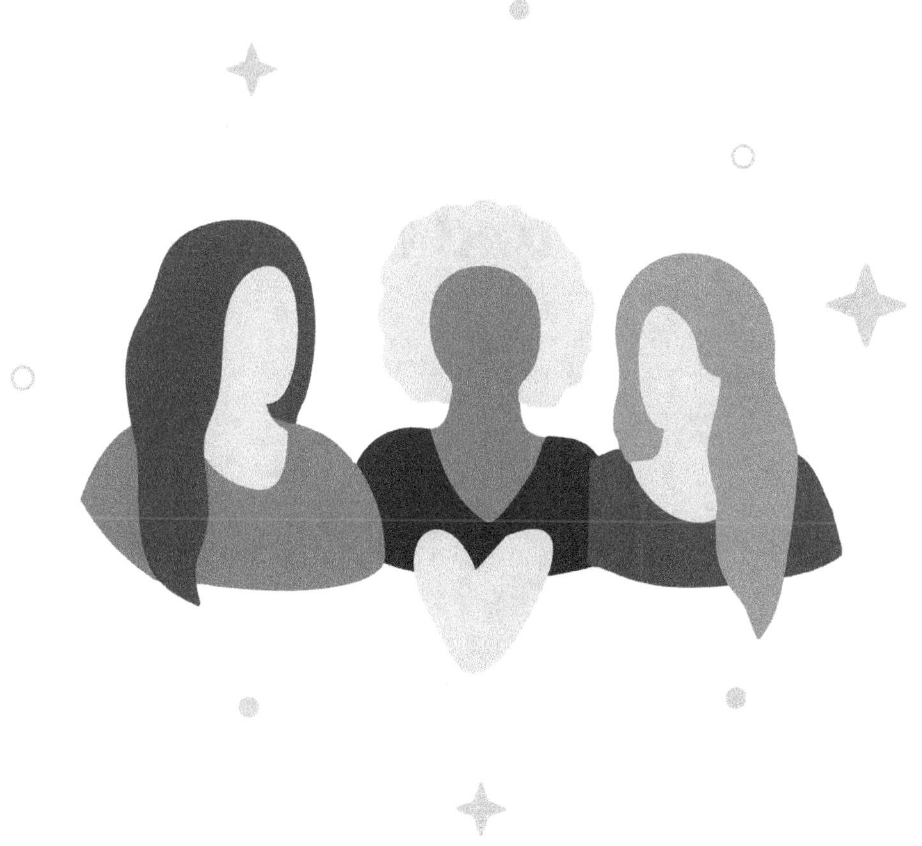

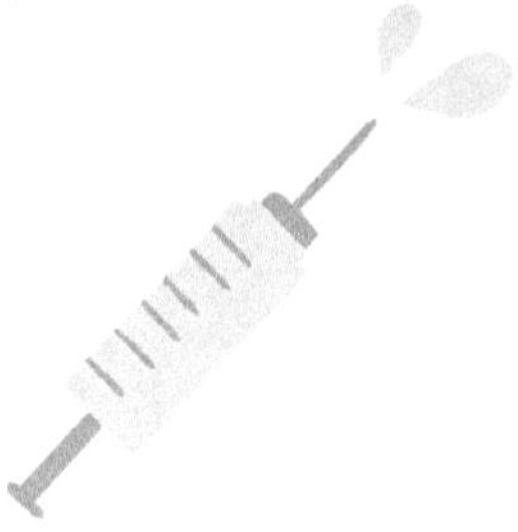

PART 5
Pediatric Healthcare and Childcare

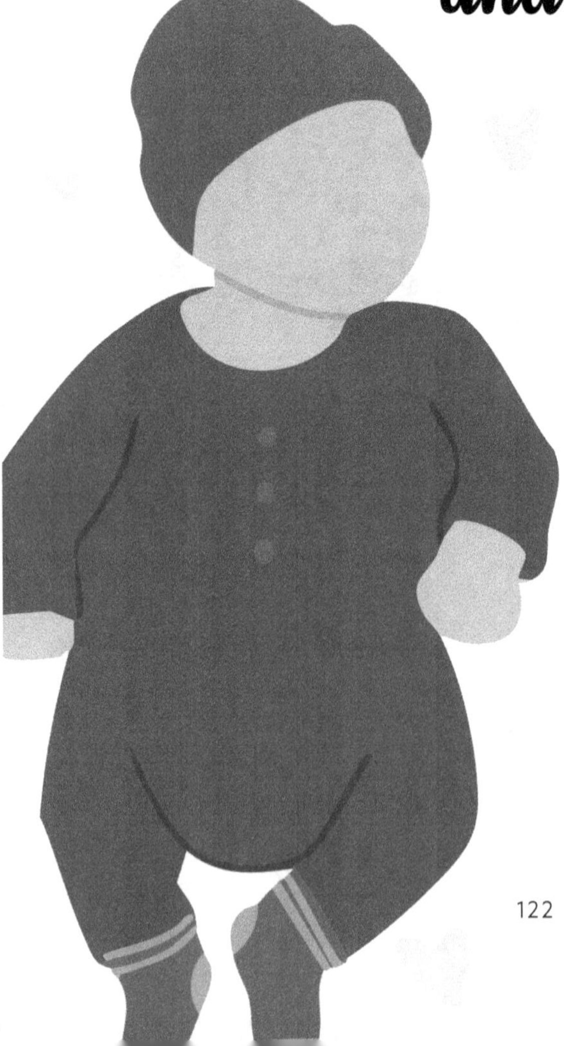

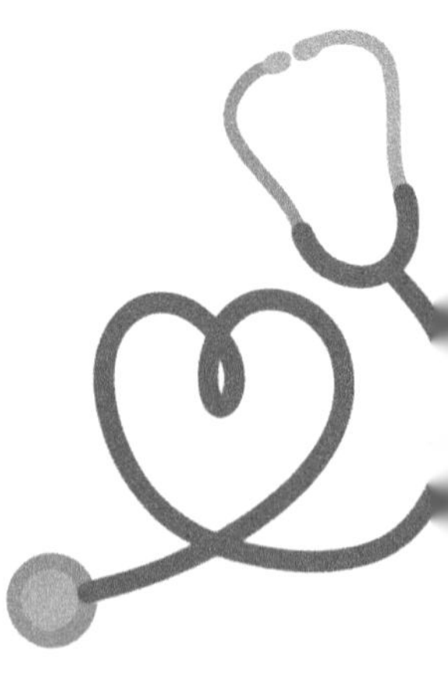

Stuffy noses are no fun at any age, are they? When we first moved to Switzerland, my daughter was barely four months old, and we were living in temporary accommodations. One night, she had a bad stuffy nose, and nothing we did seemed to work. Her breathing was laborious, and my worry started to escalate. It was the middle of the night in an unknown country, and we hadn't even been there a week.

We didn't have our trusted pediatrician working in a hospital near us. We didn't even know where the pediatric hospital was! My anxiety was compounded by the stress of the move, making me question whether we had made the right decision. But my husband, ever the calm one, dialed an emergency number he found. The people on the other end of the phone were very helpful, assisting us and even checking up on us over the next few days.

So, yes, moving to a new country can be exciting, but finding the best care for your child can be a daunting part of it. Don't worry; I've got you covered! In this chapter, I'll guide you through finding reliable **pediatric healthcare** and **childcare** options in your new home, so your child will get the best care possible.

We'll start with the basics of local healthcare systems and how to find the right providers. Then, we'll tackle the nitty-gritty of registering and keeping up with pediatric care.

Need day-care services or a babysitter? We'll explore those options too, with tips on finding and evaluating the best choices. And for those juggling work and childcare, we'll share some handy time management and self-care strategies. With the right info, you'll feel confident managing your child's healthcare and childcare needs in your new home. Let's get started!

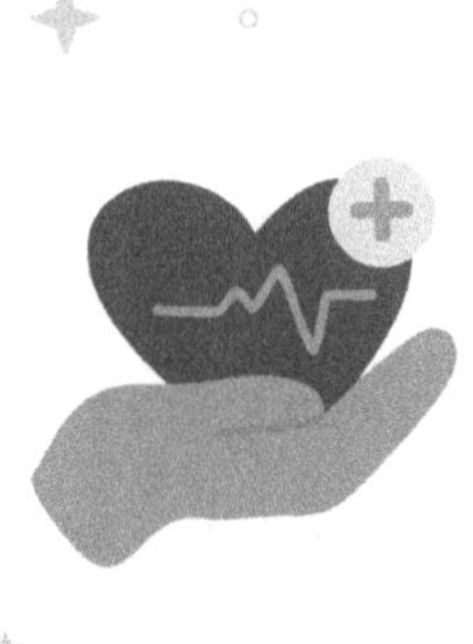

NAVIGATING THE LOCAL HEALTHCARE SYSTEM

When it comes to healthcare for kids, different parts of the world have their own way of doing things. For example, in the United States and Switzerland, pediatricians are the go-to experts for children's health, from birth through adolescence. In many European countries, though, kids might first see a general practitioner or a family doctor who handles health concerns for all ages. And in some places, especially in public health settings, nurses play a big role in routine checkups and vaccination programs. Understanding these differences can help you set the right expectations and make sure your children get the care they need

SYSTEM STRUCTURE

Understanding the healthcare system's structure in a new country is a bit like solving a puzzle, especially when it comes to pediatric care. Most developed countries have well-coordinated systems that offer various levels of care, from primary consultations to specialized treatments.

Expat parents have got to know whether the healthcare system is public, private, or a mix of both, and how its make-up affects your access to pediatric services.

Countries like the UK or Sweden offer universal access to their public healthcare model, but they could have longer wait times for non-emergency pediatric consultations. On the flip side, the USA, some Middle Eastern countries, and other places with a private healthcare system or a significant private sector component might offer quicker access to pediatric specialists, but at a higher cost.

Identifying Your Child's Healthcare Provider

CRITERIA FOR HEALTHCARE PROVIDERS

Choosing a healthcare provider for your child while living abroad involves a few important considerations that can deeply affect their well-being. Let's break it down to make it easier.

KEY FACTORS TO CONSIDER

- **Scope of Care:** Think about what services your child might need. Are you looking for routine checkups, emergency care, or specialty consultations? Make sure the provider you choose has adequate skills to offer these services.

- **Specialty:** If your child has specific health issues like allergies, asthma, or other chronic conditions, you'll want a provider who specializes in pediatrics care.

- **Accessibility:** Since this decision concerns your child's health, you must consider factors like the provider's location, their language skills (especially if you're in a non-English speaking country), and how easy it is to get appointments.

FINDING THE RIGHT FIT

Finding the right healthcare provider—a nurse, general practitioner, or pediatrician—depends largely on your child's health needs and the healthcare system of the country you're in. Here's how to make that decision:

1. **Assess Your Child's Needs:** Figure out whether your child needs routine care or has specific medical conditions that might require a pediatrician's specialized attention.

2. **Research Local Healthcare Providers:** Gather information from local expat groups, online forums, or local health authorities about the available healthcare providers. These sources can provide insights into who specializes in what, the quality of care they provide, and an overview of patients' experiences.

3. **Consider the Healthcare Framework:** In some countries, general practitioners serve as gatekeepers to specialized services. In other words, you have no choice but to start with a general practitioner. In other places, you can directly access pediatricians if your child's condition warrants it.

4. **Visit Potential Providers:** If possible, schedule a preliminary visit to see the healthcare facility, meet the provider, and discuss your child's health needs. This visit can give you a feel for whether the provider's style and approach align with your expectations. Don't hesitate to switch doctors if you're not comfortable with one—it's important to find someone you trust.

5. Language and Cultural Competence: Especially in a foreign country, finding a provider who speaks your language or understands your cultural background can improve the quality of healthcare your child receives and reduce misunderstandings.

6. Emergency Access: Consider how quickly you can access medical help in an emergency. If you think it's necessary, specifically look for providers who offer after-hours service or are affiliated with a clinic that provides comprehensive emergency services.

By carefully considering these aspects, you can make a more informed decision about which healthcare provider is the best fit for your child. The goal here is to make sure your little one receives the best possible care in your new home country.

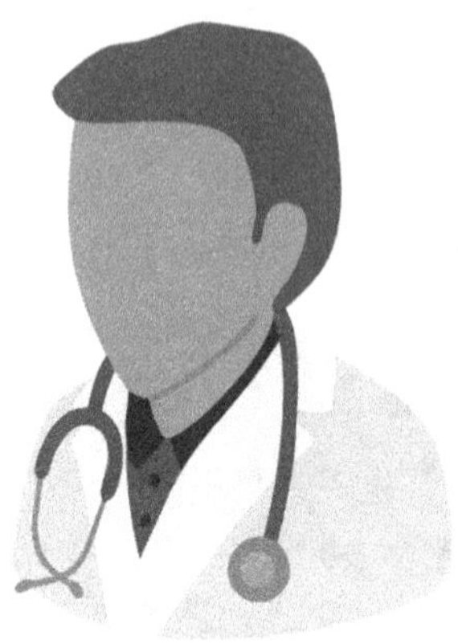

ESTABLISHING PEDIATRIC CARE

FIRST STEPS IN REGISTRATION

Worrying about your baby's health is natural; it's the motherly instinct, after all. When you move abroad, this anxiety somehow gets even worse. The first step you should take to make sure your child receives proper medical care while you're staying abroad is registering them with a local healthcare provider. It's a kind of long process, and you have to gather the required documentation, which may include your child's birth certificate, vaccination records, and any medical records you have from your home country. Then, you need to follow the exact registration procedure, which can vary widely from one country to another. In some places, you might need to register with a local health authority or directly with a clinic or hospital.

Once you have the necessary documents, the next step is the initial health assessment. This comprehensive checkup establishes a health baseline for your child. It's also an excellent opportunity for you to discuss any concerns you may have about your child's health with the provider. Be prepared to provide detailed information about your child's medical history, allergies, and any ongoing treatments.

CONTINUITY OF CARE

If your child has ongoing health needs or conditions that require regular monitoring, I don't need to tell you how important it is to ensure continuity of their care in a new country. Here are some tips to help manage this process:

1. **Transferring Medical Records:** When moving abroad, travel with a complete copy of your child's medical records. You may need to have these documents translated if they're not in your new country's language. These records should be detailed and include information about any past procedures, ongoing conditions, and medications.

2. **Setting up Initial Consultations:** The next step is to register your child with a healthcare provider in your new country and schedule an initial consultation. Use this opportunity to hand over your child's medical records and discuss his or her health comprehensively. The goal of this meeting is to make the transition process smoother for both you and your child. Discuss any complex health needs your child may have and the care they have received so far. This way, your doctor is completely informed about their needs.

3. **Developing a Care Plan:** Once the initial consultations are out of the way, work with your healthcare provider to develop a care plan that addresses both immediate health needs and longer-term medical care. This plan may include regular checkups, vaccination schedules, and referrals to specialists if needed.

4. Communication: Establish a clear line of communication with your healthcare provider. While dealing with your child's health scares can understandably cause mini heart-attacks (trust me, I've been there), you can take certain steps to decrease the stress associated with healthcare in a new environment. To begin with, find out how to reach your provider(s) in case of an emergency and understand the process for scheduling appointments or seeking advice.

5. Seek Support: If you find dealing with the local healthcare system overwhelming, consider seeking support from expatriate groups or health advocates who can offer guidance based on their experiences or professional knowledge.

When you take these steps, your child will be sure to receive consistent, reliable healthcare support, making your transition to a new country smoother for your entire family.

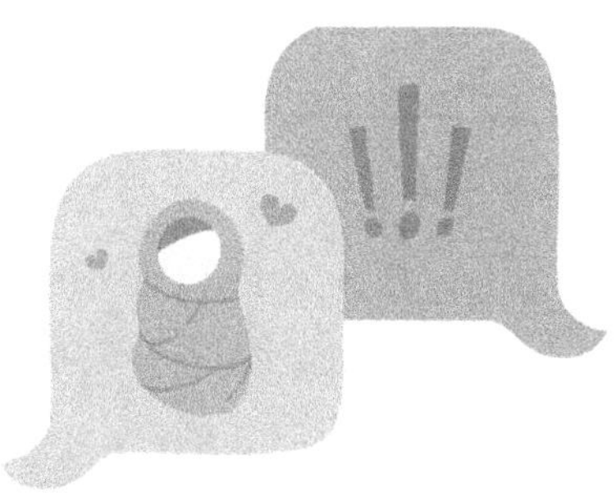

The First Trip to a Pediatrician: A Real-Life Tale

In 2016, Danielle sat next to her husband at the back of the Miami pediatric office, her fingers nervously tapping her knee. The room buzzed with the quiet chatter of other mothers and an occasional baby's cry.

They were waiting for their newborn's first appointment with their pediatrician. Back in the Brazilian Federal District, or Brasília, a doctor's appointment felt almost therapeutic—a chance to talk, to be heard, to feel reassured—and she needed that now more than ever. Not only was she new to this whole caring-for-a-baby thing, but she was also in a new country without a support network. To add to her stress, she was struggling with breastfeeding, like many mothers.

As she looked around, the sterile, personality-lacking room felt daunting. Pediatricians' offices back home were so much more inviting for children, with colorful walls, playful murals, and a toy area. Doctors put a lot of time and effort into making it feel less clinical. But this clinic's white walls and harsh fluorescent lighting made her feel even more isolated and out of place.

"Vitor," the nurse called out her baby's name, her voice cutting through Danielle's thoughts.

Danielle and her husband jumped to their feet. Her heart raced as they followed the nurse into an even smaller room. The room felt cramped, with one stool, a single chair, and an exam table taking up most of the space. The nurse quickly checked the baby. While her movements were efficient, they were devoid of warmth. Then the pediatrician entered, his demeanor professional and decisive.

He examined the baby, his hands moving swiftly and methodically. Then, almost as an afterthought, he looked up at Danielle.

"Do you have any questions?" he asked in a flat tone.

Her mind raced. She had so many questions about the baby's health, breastfeeding, and how to navigate this new life as a mother in a foreign country. But the cold, clinical environment did nothing to make her feel reassured. Instead, it added to her overwhelm. The chance for the kind of meaningful conversation she would have had back home seemed out of reach.

Her voice faltered as she tried to remember the questions she had rehearsed. "I... um...," she stammered, but nothing came out. The words she needed seemed to dissolve in the sterile air.

The pediatrician waited for a moment, then nodded curtly. "Vitor is going to need to drink formula to help him with his weight," he said, before turning to leave.

Danielle watched him go, a wave of frustration and loneliness washing over her. She looked at her husband, who squeezed her hand comfortingly. This wasn't the supportive, encouraging experience for which she'd hoped, but she knew she had to find a way to make her way through this new world, for her baby's sake.

Determined to make the best of her situation, Danielle decided to take proactive steps. From that day forward, she prepared a list of questions for each appointment, covering all her concerns despite the brief and impersonal consultations. She also started reaching out to local expat communities online, seeking advice and support from other mothers who had faced similar challenges.

Soon, Danielle began to adapt. She found ways to blend her expectations with the realities of her new environment, learning to advocate for herself and her child. Through persistence and the help of her husband and newfound friends, she gradually built a network that provided the emotional and practical support she needed.

Her experience highlights the importance of preparation and self-advocacy for mothers living abroad as they're finding their way in unfamiliar healthcare systems. Although the process may be challenging, discovering ways to connect and seek support can make all the difference in the well-being of both mother and child.

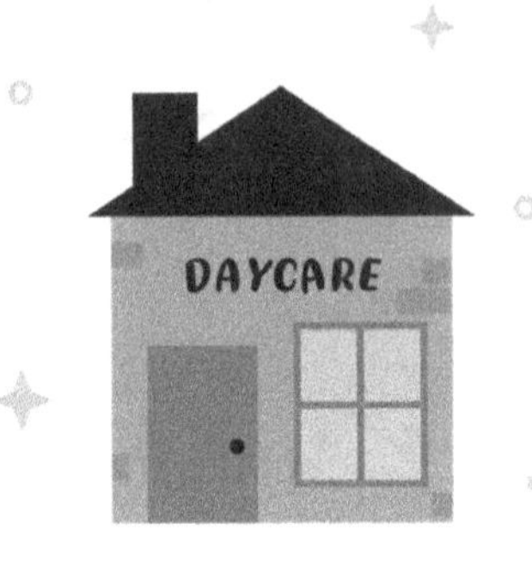

DAYCARE, BABYSITTING, AND SUPPORT SERVICES FOR PARENTS ABROAD

For parents around the globe, finding reliable childcare is a critical concern. But it becomes even more challenging when you're living and working abroad. Whether you need to return to work, run errands, or simply take a break, knowing your child is in good hands gives you much-needed peace of mind.

As a foreign national, be prepared to face unique difficulties in figuring out childcare. You might be unfamiliar with the **types of daycare** facilities available, the cultural expectations around **babysitting**, or even how to find a trustworthy **nanny** or **au pair**. On top of this challenge, language barriers and different regulatory standards can make things even more complicated.

But don't worry! This part of the chapter will guide you through the maze of daycare and babysitting services in your new home country. From understanding the different types of available childcare to the importance of licensing, we'll cover everything you need to know to make informed decisions. We'll also look at several practical tips on finding and vetting providers, so you can make the best decision for your family.

Additionally, we'll explore **other support options**, like parent co-ops and playgroups, and provide strategies for balancing work and childcare. And, to make it all more relatable, we'll share a real-life story from a parent who successfully conquered these challenges.

So, let's get you prepared to find the best care for your little one in your new environment.

UNDERSTANDING AND FINDING DAYCARE SERVICES

Finding the right daycare facility in a new country can feel overwhelming. A lot of questions and concerns may slow down your decision-making process, and you may even begin wondering whether the stress of finding a good daycare is worth it. But with a bit of guidance, you'll find the perfect place for your little one. Let's explore some tips and tricks to make the process easier (and maybe even fun)! First up, let's talk about the different types of daycare facilities that are generally available.

In a new country, parents often face initial hesitations about putting their kids in daycare, especially when the way things are done there starkly contrasts with what they're used to back home. Debora's experience is a perfect example. She shared, "Gabi ended up going to daycare at one-and-a-half-years old, and for me, this part was very difficult. It felt like I had a bit of a block with this daycare thing, you know? I would visit daycares, and I had an idea of what a daycare should be like based on my experience in Brazil. But in New Zealand, things are more relaxed. They have a culture of allowing the child to do what comes naturally to them. For example, I'd see a child climbing something and think it was dangerous, but the daycare staff would say, 'How wonderful, look at that development!' I had to accept it because I needed to work. The first few weeks were tough, and I was very worried, but then I saw that it was so good for her. Despite everything, by the end of the day, she was happy, safe, and well-fed."

Debora's story demonstrates the common concerns parents might have about safety and how educational philosophies between countries may be very different. These differences can lead to some hesitation in opting for these services. However, with time, many parents find that their children adapt well and even thrive in these new environments. The key is to understand the types of daycare facilities available in your new country and find one that aligns as closely as possible with your values and expectations.

Public Daycare

- **Benefits:** Usually more affordable due to government subsidies and provides a structured environment.

- **Drawbacks:** Might have longer waiting lists and less flexible hours.

- **Costs:** Usually free or costs less than other options, but it can vary based on income and eligibility for subsidies.

Private Daycare

- **Benefits:** More flexible hours, smaller groups, and possibly more activities.

- **Drawbacks:** Despite being private, some still have waitlists. In some cases, parents have to register before the baby is born to secure a spot.

- **Costs:** High cost, depending on the services and location.

In-Home Daycare or Family Daycare

- **Benefits:** Cozier, smaller groups and a home-like setting.

- **Drawbacks:** Less regulated, so the quality can vary.

- **Costs:** Middle range, but it really depends on the provider.

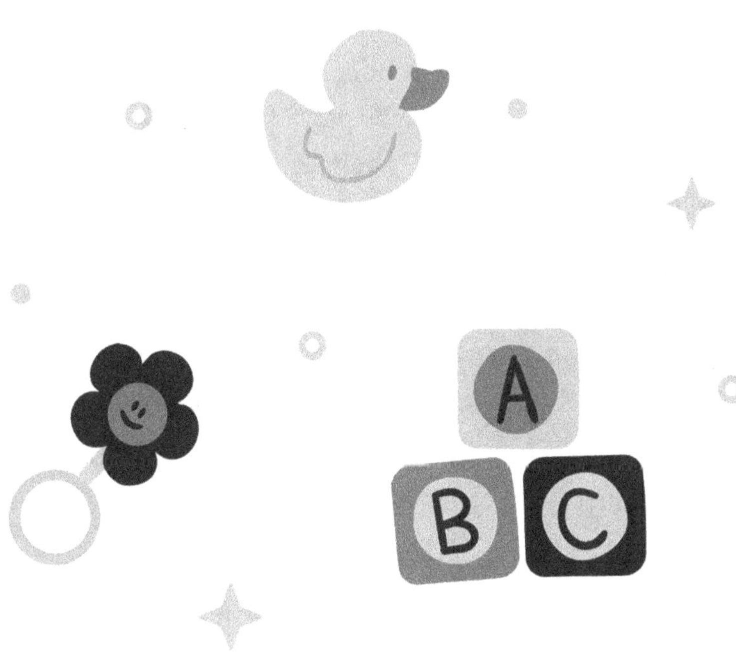

What about finding a daycare with your own cultural background as its backbone? If that possibility excites you, I'm happy to inform you that those exist too! If you happen to find one nearby, it could be the perfect fit for your child. Why not explore this option?

Take the story of Maite Furuiti's family daycare as an example. An expatriate mother living in Australia drew from her work experience in local daycares and her desire to create the best environment for her three-month-old daughter. She decided to open her own family daycare to incorporate her native language and cultural warmth into her child's life.

Years later, with many children under her care, Maite shares her unique experience: "I think of the children as part of my family. Because you get to know them so well and most of them live so close, you run into them on the street or at the supermarket. It's like they are also my kids."

Make sure the daycare facility you choose is licensed and accredited, for your child's safety and your peace of mind. Check local government websites for online databases where you can verify a daycare's licensing status and look for stamps of approval from recognized accreditation organizations. Parent reviews and recommendations can also provide valuable insights into a daycare's reputation.

By understanding the types of daycare facilities available and doing thorough research, you can find a daycare that meets your child's needs and gives you needed assurance.

VISITING AND EVALUATING DAYCARE CENTERS

When you're checking out daycare centers, find a place that feels right and in which you feel a sense of confidence. Here's what to keep an eye on:

- **First, make sure the place is clean and safe.** The space should be tidy and child-proofed, with plenty of caregivers to ensure each child gets enough attention. Trust your gut about the overall vibe—does it feel welcoming and positive?

- **When you chat with the staff, don't be shy.** Ask as many questions as you need. Ask how many children each caregiver looks after and what qualifications those caregivers have. Get a sense of what a typical day looks like and inquire about their procedures for handling emergencies and caring for sick children. You'll also need to understand their approach to discipline to make sure it's in line with your own parenting style.

- **Spend some time observing the environment and interactions.** Watch how the staff engages with the kids. Obviously, you want to see warm, positive, and engaging interactions; anything that deviates from that atmosphere may not be the best option. Notice how the children respond to the caregivers and the overall atmosphere. Are the kids happy and relaxed? These observations can give you a real sense of how your child will feel in this new environment.

Before we talk about babysitting services, let me share a golden nugget of advice I received from an American mom I once met (apologies for not remembering her name): Call the daycare as soon as possible to get a rough idea about the waiting list. And if you're from a country where waiting lists for daycare are unheard of, let me tell you—they are very real. In some places, you need to get your name on the list as soon as you find out you're having a baby. Did that pregnancy test turn up positive? Get your name on the list right away.

When I moved to Switzerland over a year ago, I had no idea the wait would be so long just to secure a couple of half-days at a daycare. Thankfully, my husband can support us while I stay at home with our little one, but this is definitely something you need to plan for, especially if you intend on heading back to work soon.

BABYSITTING SERVICES

Alright, let's talk babysitting—a true lifeline when you need a break, a night out, or just an extra hand.

Finding a Babysitter

Finding the right babysitter can be tough, but with a good strategy, you'll find that perfect match. Luana Messias, a Brazilian mother living in Kingscliff, Australia, decided to go back to work a while after the birth of her baby. She got a nanny for her youngest when she was only fifteen months old, and she shared the reasons that went into making that particular decision. "I chose to go with a nanny because I really wanted more personal care. The nanny was also Brazilian, so I thought it would be cool to have that same culture and also help teach them Kailani Portuguese. It's much more complex to try to keep the second language fluent when I enter the house. No matter how hard I try, English ends up being predominant. So having that person at home helps."

If babysitting is a service you'll need, you should start by exploring various avenues. Agencies and online platforms are great places to begin, with websites or local equivalents offering many options. Don't underestimate the power of local recommendations either. Sometimes, the best suggestions come from people you trust—fellow non-native parents, neighbors, or your colleagues might know of a reliable babysitter who understands the local customs and your family's needs. Of course, community boards and social media can be treasure troves of information, with listings and recommendations often posted in local Facebook groups (yeah, Facebook is still a thing!) or other online communities.

When searching for a good babysitter, here are some factors you should consider:

- **Experience and References:** Look for a babysitter with experience and glowing references. It's always good to hear from other parents about what they've seen. Knowing that others have had positive experiences can help you feel more confident about your choice.

- **First Aid and CPR Certification:** It's important to have a babysitter who knows first aid and CPR, so they can handle emergencies capably. If your babysitter doesn't have these certifications yet, consider whether you might be willing to pay for them to undergo this training. Sometimes, nannies might not have the money to afford these courses, but having them do it is an investment in your child's safety. Offering to cover the cost can help you feel secure.

- **Communication Skills**: Never underestimate the power of good communication skills! A babysitter should be able to communicate clearly with both you and your child.

- **Patience and Reliability**: Patience is an enormous part of dealing with children. Additionally, the babysitter should be reliable and punctual.

- **Compatibility with Your Family**: The babysitter should fit well with your family's dynamics and values. A trial run can help determine this compatibility.

- **Background Checks**: Consider running a background check for additional reassurance. Many agencies and online platforms offer this service.

- **Local Knowledge**: A babysitter who understands local customs and knows the area can be a great asset, especially in case of an emergency or when planning activities.

By prioritizing these traits, you'll find a babysitter who meets your family's needs and provides a safe, nurturing environment for your child.

Interviewing Potential Babysitters

Once you've shortlisted a few candidates, it's time to get to know them better. An interview is really just a friendly chat to see if an applicant is a good fit for your family. Ask them about their experience handling children in the same age group as your child, and don't shy away from asking for references from past babysitting jobs. You should also know how they handle emergencies or unexpected situations and what activities they enjoy doing with kids. Additionally, observe how your child reacts around them. It might be easier to tell when the child is a bit older, but it's important to listen to your child if they seem uncomfortable with someone. Watch out for red flags like vague answers about their experience or hesitation in providing references, as these can be indicators that they might not be the right fit. Remember, even though you can keep it friendly and casual, this is a job interview—take it seriously. Parents should feel comfortable asking all the necessary questions, as they will be entrusting this person with the most important part of their lives.

Red Flags to Watch For:

- **Vague Answers**: If a babysitter gives vague or unclear answers about their experience, it could be a sign they're not being completely honest.

- **Hesitation with References**: Hesitation about or inability to provide references is a major red flag.

- **Negative Reviews**: Check online reviews or ask around. Consistent negative feedback is obviously a bad sign.

- **Unreliable Communication**: If they are difficult to reach or communicate poorly, it might indicate future reliability issues.

- **Unprofessional Behavior**: Arriving late to interviews, being unprepared, or displaying unprofessional behavior should raise concerns.

- **Discomfort with Your Child**: Trust your child's instincts as well. If he or she seems uncomfortable around the babysitter, you might want to reconsider.

By watching out for these red flags, you'll be better equipped to find a babysitter who meets your family's needs and provides a safe, nurturing environment for your child.

Conducting Background Checks and Verifying References

Don't skip this step—it's essential to put your mind at ease about your child's safety. Many agencies and online platforms provide background checks, but if you're hiring independently, ask the babysitter if they underwent a background check recently or how you can obtain one. Calling their references is also a must. Ask questions like, "How did your children feel about the babysitter?" and "Did you have any issues or concerns?" to get a clear picture of their reliability and compatibility with your family.

ENSURING A CULTURAL FIT

When hiring a babysitter abroad, it can take time to find someone who understands and respects your family's cultural background and language. But with some effort, you'll get there. Make sure they're aware of any cultural practices or dietary restrictions you follow, as this makes a big difference in creating a comfortable environment for your child. Language skills are equally important. If your child is more comfortable speaking a certain language, ensure the babysitter can communicate effectively in that language.

TRAINING AND INTEGRATING THE BABYSITTER INTO YOUR HOUSEHOLD

Once you've selected a babysitter, help them understand your family's routines and expectations. Spend the first few sessions together, showing them around, explaining routines, and introducing them to your child's favorite activities and toys. Make sure the babysitter knows where to find emergency contact numbers, first aid supplies, and any specific medical information about your child. Establish a system for checking in and providing feedback, whether it's a daily log of activities or regular check-ins. Open communication will keep everything running smoothly.

Alternative Childcare Options and Planning for Emergencies

Now that we've figured out how to go about picking the right babysitter or daycare facility for you and your baby, let's talk about those times when these traditional solutions just don't fit the bill. Maybe your schedule is unpredictable, or you just need a bit of extra help every now and then. No matter the situation, it's wise to have a few backup childcare options and a reliable emergency plan. Let's get started.

EXPLORING ALTERNATIVE CHILDCARE OPTIONS

One fantastic option is joining a parent co-op. This is like a friendly neighborhood club where parents take turns looking after each other's kids. It's not only a great way to save on childcare costs; it's also an excellent opportunity to build a community. Having a group of parents who understand your challenges and can step in to help out is definitely a blessing. Plus, your kids get to make new friends and playmates, and so do you!

Parent co-ops are common in many places around the world, such as the United States, Canada, the UK, Australia, and Germany. By joining a co-op, you can find affordable childcare and build a supportive network of friends. It's a win-win for everyone involved!

Another option is drop-in centers. These are the magic wand or "easy button" of childcare—you can drop your kids off for a few hours while you run errands, go to appointments, or just take some much-needed me time. These centers keep your kids safe and entertained, with trained staff and fun activities. Typically, you book these places online and pay by the hour.

Playgroups are also fantastic! While your child socializes with children in their age group, you can take a quick break. These groups often meet weekly and are a great way for your kids to interact with others while you connect with fellow parents. Look for local community centers, libraries, or expat groups that organize such gatherings.

Planning for Emergencies

Now, let's chat about planning for those unexpected moments when you need childcare in a pinch. Because let's face it—emergencies don't warn us well in advance. Basically, you need a backup plan for your backup plan.

First, create a list of emergency contacts. These could be trusted friends, neighbors, or family members who live nearby. Make sure these people are aware they're on your list and are comfortable stepping in if needed. It's always good to have a mix of people who can cover different times of the day or different types of emergencies.

Next, look into emergency childcare services in your area. Some daycare centers and agencies offer last-minute or drop-in care specifically for emergencies. It's worth knowing who these providers are and what their protocols are before you find yourself in a bind. However, do your research long before an emergency knocks on your door, so you don't have to use up your time when things are already chaotic.

You should also consider preparing an emergency go-bag for your child. A go-bag is a mini survival kit with everything your child might need if you have to drop them off with someone else unexpectedly. Pack it with things like diapers, wipes, a change of clothes, snacks, and comfort items like a favorite toy or blanket. This way, if you have to hand your child over quickly, everything they need is already set to go.

Finally, don't forget about online resources. Many apps and websites can connect you with emergency babysitters on short notice. It's a good idea to sign up for a few of these services ahead of time, so you're not scrambling to create an account when you're in urgent need.

Making It All Work

By combining these alternative childcare options with a solid emergency plan, you can make it through the ups and downs of motherhood in a foreign country with a little more confidence and a lot less stress. Remember, preparation and building a supportive network are the name of the game. Whether it's a co-op, a drop-in center, or a list of reliable emergency contacts, these options might just make all the difference when you need them most.

Managing childcare in a foreign country doesn't have to be a solo enterprise. With the right mix of resources and a proactive approach, you'll find the perfect balance between handling your outside responsibilities and looking after your most important priority—your child. And who knows, along the way, you might even make some great friends and create a strong support network that lasts a lifetime.

Balancing Work and Childcare

Finding the balance between work and childcare can feel like juggling flaming torches while riding a unicycle. It's challenging, but when you do it right, it can also be incredibly rewarding. So, let's look at some practical tips that can make this balancing act a little less daunting.

- **Time management is your best friend:** Create a flexible schedule that accommodates both your professional responsibilities and your child's needs. It's like creating the perfect recipe—you need the right ingredients in the right amounts at the right times. Start by setting clear boundaries for work and family time. When you're working, focus on work. When you're with your child, be fully present. Easier said than done, right? I know; this is something I struggle with too. But with practice, it becomes more manageable.

- **Utilizing technology can also be a game-changer:** Tools like shared calendars, task management apps, and even simple reminders can help keep you on track. For instance, if you know you have a big project deadline coming up, plan your child's activities so that he or she will be entertained while you focus.

- **Speaking of keeping kids entertained, don't underestimate the power of planning engaging activities.** A well-timed playdate, a creative craft project, or even a favorite movie can buy you some precious uninterrupted work time. But don't just focus on keeping them busy—find a way to make sure they're having fun and learning while you're getting things done.

- **Flexible work arrangements can be a lifesaver for many parents.** If your job allows it, explore options like remote work, flexible hours, or even a compressed workweek. These arrangements can give you the breathing room you need to manage both work and childcare more effectively. Don't be shy about discussing these options with your employer! More companies are recognizing the importance of work-life balance these days, so your boss may be more accommodating than you'd expect.

- **Self-care is another important component of balancing work and childcare.** It's easy to get caught up in the hustle and forget to take care of yourself, but burnout helps no one. Signs of burnout include constant fatigue, irritability, and feeling overwhelmed. Make sure to schedule some "me time" into your week, whether it's a quiet cup of coffee in the morning, a quick workout, or a few minutes of meditation. If these feelings persist, don't hesitate to speak with a specialist. Taking care of your mental and physical health will help you become a more patient and effective parent and employee.

- **Connecting with a support network can also make a world of difference.** Reach out to fellow expat parents, join local community groups, or participate in online forums. Sharing experiences and advice can provide valuable insights and a sense of camaraderie. Sometimes, just knowing you're not alone in this juggling act can be incredibly reassuring.

- **And finally, don't forget to celebrate the small victories.** Managed to get through a conference call without any interruptions? Great job, mama! Made it to your child's school event without feeling rushed? Perfect! These moments are worth acknowledging. Balancing work and childcare is an ongoing process, and every little win counts.

In the end, finding the right balance is a mix of flexibility, creativity, and a lot of patience. Structured planning with a bit of improvisation can help you create a routine that works for both your career and your family life. And remember, it's okay to ask for help and adjust your approach as needed. With time and practice, you'll find a rhythm that allows you to flourish in both roles.

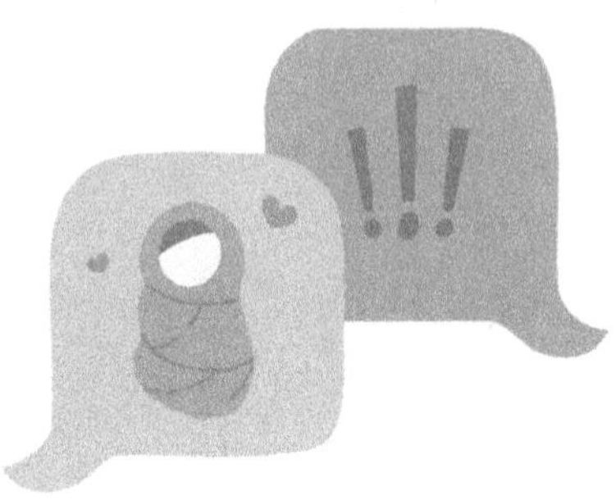

A French Daycare Saga: A Real-Life Tale

Drika Muniz stood in the small, cluttered kitchen of her Parisian apartment, white-knuckling her phone. The apartment felt cramped, suffocating even, with baby toys strewn everywhere and the constant hum of city life filtering through the thin walls. Drika and her partner Julien had been dreaming of more space, more freedom, and perhaps a little more sunshine.

They had talked endlessly about moving to Nice, where the pace of life was slower and the rent was cheaper. With Julien working from home and Drika's extended maternity leave nearing its end, the pressure to make a decision was mounting. The impossibility of finding a daycare spot in Paris had pushed Drika to the edge. As someone who worked in daycare herself, she knew her only real shot at securing a spot for their son was if she returned to work. And while working in daycare wasn't her dream, if she had to go back, it might as well be in a place she liked.

She longed for a place that was more open—maybe somewhere they could have both the vibrancy of city life and the tranquility of more spacious surroundings. Nice seemed like the perfect compromise, offering both the cultural richness they cherished and the open, sunny spaces they craved.

Without saying anything to Julien, Drika took a deep breath and called her boss to find out if the Nice branch had a place for her. Her heart pounded with each ring. The phone clicked, and a friendly voice greeted her on the other end. Drika quickly explained their situation, trying to keep her voice steady despite the anxiety bubbling up inside her.

"Yes, of course, we have a spot for your baby," her boss said. "And, actually, we have a position open for you as well."

Drika's breath caught in her throat. Could it really be this simple? She thanked her boss several times, hung up the phone, and felt a wave of relief wash over her.

That evening, over a bottle of wine, Drika shared the news with Julien. "They have a spot for the baby and a job for me," she said, her voice trembling.

Julien looked up, his eyes wide with surprise. "You're kidding. That's incredible!"

They sat down together, the enormity of the decision ahead of them settling in. It was a choice between staying in Paris, struggling with high rents and no daycare, or moving to Nice, where benefits like accessible childcare and open spaces beckoned them.

For the next two days, they worked tirelessly, contacting numerous landlords both day and night. Visiting Nice for every viewing was impractical, so they scheduled a video call for a virtual tour of a promising apartment. Two days after that video visit, they finalized the contract.

A week later, their decision was made. They packed up their small apartment, sold what they couldn't take, and set off for Nice. As they drove away from Paris, Drika felt a sense of liberation she hadn't expected. They were starting from scratch, but with the promise of a better life for their family.

Arriving in Nice, they were welcomed by the gentle sea breeze and the Mediterranean Sea's azure waters. Their new apartment, just a stone's throw from the beach, felt like a dream come true. The daycare was everything they had hoped for, and Drika quickly settled into her new job.

Looking out over the sparkling sea, Drika knew they had made the right choice. They had traded the hustle and bustle of Paris for the tranquility of the Riviera, and their family was thriving. It was a fresh start, a new adventure, and most importantly, they were in this together.

Sometimes, taking a risk and making that first move is necessary. Being open to new changes and embracing where they might lead can bring unexpected joy and fulfillment. Drika's story is a testament to the beauty of new beginnings and the hope that comes with embracing life's adventures.

Summary of Key Points

NAVIGATING THE LOCAL HEALTHCARE SYSTEM

- **Know the Key Players**: Figuring out if your kid needs a pediatrician, a general practitioner, or a nurse is like choosing between multiple answers without knowing the exact question. Get to know who's who in your new country.

- **Get Registered Early**: Register with a local healthcare provider as soon as possible to avoid any surprises.

- **Understand the System**: Understanding your new home's healthcare system, whether it's public, private, or a mix, will help you avoid unexpected bureaucratic hurdles.

IDENTIFYING YOUR CHILD'S HEALTHCARE PROVIDER

- **Assess Needs**: Determine whether your child requires routine check-ups or specialized care.

- **Research Local Providers**: Use expat groups and online forums to find the healthcare providers everyone's raving about (or criticizing mercilessly).

- **Check Accessibility**: Make sure the provider's office isn't located in the next time zone and they speak a language you understand (both literally and figuratively).

ESTABLISHING PEDIATRIC CARE

- **Gather Documents**: Have birth certificates, vaccination records, and medical histories ready.

- **Continuity of Care**: Transfer medical records and set up initial consultations to get everyone on the same page.

- **Communication is Key**: Ensure you have an easy way to contact your healthcare provider(s). Being able to reach them when needed can make all the difference in managing your child's health and well-being.

DAYCARE, BABYSITTING, AND SUPPORT SERVICES FOR PARENTS ABROAD

- **Understand Types of Daycare Available**: Public, private, or in-home daycare—each has its perks and quirks.

- **Evaluate Options**: Visit centers, ask questions, and watch how the staff interacts with kids. Make sure it feels right.

- **Find Babysitters**: Use agencies, recommendations, and online platforms. Do a thorough background check and ensure your babysitter gets your family's vibe.

- **Explore Alternatives**: Parent co-ops, drop-in centers, and playgroups can be lifesavers.

BALANCING WORK AND CHILDCARE

- **Time Management**: Create a schedule that works for both your job and your little one(s).

- **Utilize Technology**: Use apps and tools to stay organized and keep track of everyone's schedule. If you use them efficiently, it's like having a personal assistant who never asks for a coffee break.

- **Self-Care**: Don't forget to take some time for yourself. Even superheroes need their downtime.

- **Connect with Others**: Join local community groups or online forums.

By keeping these key points in mind, you can approach pediatric healthcare and childcare with confidence in your new country, making the process easier for both you and your little ones. Who knew moving abroad could be this much fun?

CONCLUSION

As we come to the end of this book, it's clear that embracing maternity abroad is a complex, challenging, and ultimately rewarding endeavor. From the initial culture shock and the quest for quality healthcare to the joys of bringing your baby to this world, you have an exciting adventure ahead. The stories shared throughout this book paint a vivid picture of the resilience, adaptability, and love that define the experience of motherhood abroad.

ENCOURAGING FUTURE FOREIGN MOTHERS

For those considering the path of motherhood abroad, the stories and insights shared in this book offer both inspiration and practical guidance. While the prospect of handling pregnancy, childbirth, and parenting in a foreign country can be intimidating, it is also an incredible opportunity for personal and family growth.

To future expatriate mothers, we offer these words of encouragement:

1. **Embrace the adventure:** Approach the path of motherhood abroad with an open mind, a sense of curiosity, and a willingness to step outside your comfort zone. Embrace the challenges as opportunities for growth and learning, and trust in your ability to adapt and bloom.[26]

2. **Build a support network:** As demonstrated by several stories in this book, having a strong support system is a must for international mothers. Seek out local expat communities, join online forums and groups, and don't be afraid to reach out for help when you need it. Remember, you are not alone in this journey.[26]

3. Celebrate your cultural identity: Living abroad offers a unique opportunity to reflect on and celebrate your cultural heritage. Find ways to incorporate your traditions, language, and values into your family life, while also embracing the richness of your host culture. Your children will benefit from growing up with a strong sense of cultural identity and an appreciation for diversity.[26]

4. Prioritize self-care: Motherhood is demanding under any circumstances, but the challenges of parenting abroad can be especially taxing. Make self-care a priority, whether that means carving out time for hobbies and relaxation, seeking professional support when needed, or simply being kind and patient with yourself. Remember, taking care of yourself is an essential part of taking care of your family.[26]

A Final Note

Hey there, fellow adventurers in motherhood!

As we wrap up, I just want to take a moment to acknowledge the incredible journey you're on. Dealing with maternity abroad is no small feat. In fact, it's a rollercoaster of challenges and triumphs, of personal growth and family adventures, and of bridging cultures and building global communities.

To all the amazing international moms who shared their stories and insights in this book, thank you from the bottom of my heart. Your experiences inspire and guide those who are following in your footsteps.

And to the future non-native moms who are just starting out, embrace the journey! Trust your strength and remember that you're part of a global sisterhood of women who are changing the world, one family at a time.

Let's go forward together, as a community of mothers, supporting and learning from each other and celebrating the incredible journey of motherhood across borders. Together, we can create a world where all children grow up as global citizens, rooted in love, diversity, and cultural understanding.

APPENDIX

Welcome to the appendix, your handy guide to approaching motherhood in a new country. Consider this a comprehensive checklist—a practical tool for anyone looking to move and settle abroad who hopes to become a parent eventually. Plus, it has a glossary of essential maternity and healthcare terms in multiple languages—because let's face it, understanding medical jargon in a foreign language can be tricky. And to top it off, I've included insights from interviews with experts. It's all here to make your journey a bit smoother and a lot more manageable.

Checklist for Expectant Mothers Moving Abroad

Preparing for a move abroad can be overwhelming, especially when you're also dealing with the joys and challenges of pregnancy. This checklist is designed to help you stay organized and ensure a smooth transition for you and your growing family.

- ☑ **Research your destination:** Learn about your new home country's culture, customs, and living conditions. Familiarize yourself with the local healthcare system, maternity leave policies, and childcare options.

- ☑ **Arrange for healthcare:** Find a reputable obstetrician or midwife in your new location, and schedule your first prenatal appointment. Make sure to transfer your medical records and any necessary prescriptions.

- ☑ **Secure housing:** Find a safe, comfortable living space that meets your family's needs. Consider factors such as proximity to healthcare facilities, schools, and other amenities that a pregnant woman, a new mom, or a toddler might need. Depending on your job, housing might be provided or subsidized, so check with your employer to learn about the options available to you. This perk can greatly ease the transition and help you settle in more smoothly.

☑ **Organize important documents:** Gather and make copies of essential documents like passports, birth certificates, marriage licenses, and medical records. Check visa and residency requirements for your new country.

☑ **Learn the language:** If you're moving to a country where they speak a different language than you, start learning basic phrases related to pregnancy and childbirth. Consider enrolling in language classes or using language learning apps.

☑ **Connect with other foreign mothers:** Reach out to international communities and online forums to connect with other mothers who have experience giving birth and raising children abroad. Their insights and support can be invaluable.

☑ **Pack wisely:** Make a list of items essential for your pregnancy and your baby's first few months. When doing so, it's a good idea to check whether the items are available in your new country. If not, you'll need to buy and carry them with you. Don't forget to pack any sentimental or cultural items that will help you feel connected to your roots.

☑ **Take care of yourself:** Prioritize self-care during this time of transition. Make time for rest, relaxation, and activities that bring you joy and help you manage stress.

☑ **Embrace the adventure:** Remember that though moving abroad during pregnancy can be challenging, it's also an incredible opportunity for personal growth and family bonding. Approach the experience with an open mind and a sense of curiosity.

Glossary of Terms Related to Maternity and Healthcare in Multiple Languages

Understanding the language of healthcare and maternity in a foreign country can be challenging. This glossary provides translations of essential terms in several common languages to help you communicate effectively with healthcare providers and support networks.

English	Spanish	Portuguese	French	German
Pregnancy	Embarazo	Gravidez	Grossesse	Schwangerschaft
Midwife	Matrona	Parteira	Sage-femme	Hebamme
Doula	Doula	Doula	Doula	Doula
Prenatal	Prenatal	Pré-natal	Prénatal	Vorgeburtlich
Ultrasound	Ultrasonido	Ultrassom	Échographie	Ultraschall
Labor	Parto	Trabalho de parto	Accouchement	Geburt
Cesarean	Cesárea	Cesariana	Césarienne	Kaiserschnitt
Breastfeeding	Lactancia	Amamentação	Allaitement	Stillen
Postpartum	Postparto	Pós-parto	Postpartum	Wochenbett
Pediatrician	Pediatra	Pediatra	Pédiatre	Kinderarzt

Remember, even with language barriers, you can always find ways to communicate and connect.

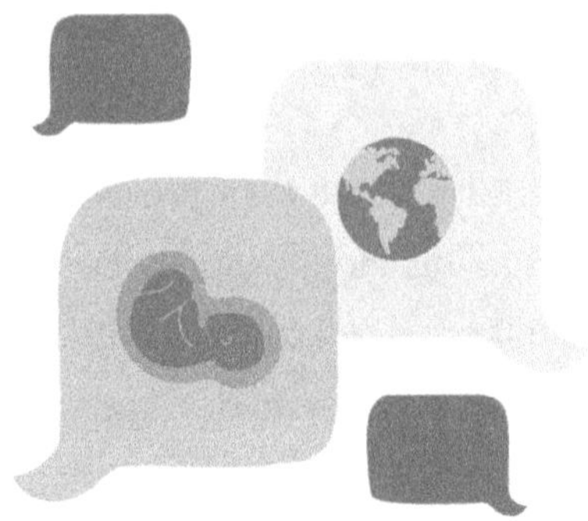

Interviews with Experts

To provide further insight and guidance for foreign mothers, I reached out to experts around the globe who are well-versed with this topic. Their perspectives offer valuable advice for handling the unique challenges and joys of maternity abroad.

FERNANDA BENGHI MARFIL | DOULA

Q. How do you adapt your support and services for mothers giving birth in a foreign country, especially when cultural practices and medical systems differ from their home country?

A. To adapt my support and services for mothers giving birth in a foreign country, I focus on each woman's specific needs, which can be diverse and unpredictable. I create a safe space by keeping an open ear and striving to maintain a non-judgmental dialogue. This space allows us to build her experience together, using her personalized information and creating a support network with other professionals as needed.

Q. Can you share insights on adapting to local postpartum practices and customs and how new mothers can blend them with their own traditions to create a comfortable and supportive environment?

A. Local postpartum practices and customs can be harmonized with a new mother's own traditions through non-judgmental support and when the people caring for her deeply understand her dreams, fears, and expectations. When a woman feels secure and embraced in her motherhood, she can confidently decide what to retain from her own culture and what to embrace from the local culture, always based on her own needs rather than external judgments.

Q. What are some key tips you can offer for working with local healthcare systems in a new country, particularly for prenatal and postnatal care?

A. It's essential to communicate openly with healthcare professionals and seek clarifications when needed. Understand that while they are the experts, you need to prioritize your comfort and security. If you aren't fluent in the local language or feel like you can't express yourself as you would like, seek support in your native language. You can even opt for online resources, including professionals who understand the migration process and are well-versed in your native tongue. Another key tip is not to feel alone on this "journey." Build a support network with other expatriates, local mother groups, and professionals who understand your cultural and linguistic needs.

SELMA VEQUI | PRENATAL VINYASA YOGA TEACHER

Q. What are the primary benefits of practicing prenatal yoga during pregnancy?

A. Prenatal Vinyasa Yoga allows the student to dive deep into her pregnant body. By connecting breath with movement, she will build up strength and stamina, and embark on a journey of self-discovery and self-care. She'll learn tools to find comfort in her body while being strong and keeping her heart open. Yoga strengthens her connection with her body and baby. She'll feel more confident and prepared for labor and parenthood. And lastly, regular practice will promote an easier recovery from pregnancy and childbirth.

Q. How can prenatal yoga help prepare expectant mothers for labor and delivery?

A. Yoga helps improve fetal positioning. Postures like downward-facing dog, extended side angle, warrior poses, and many others help lengthen the uterine ligaments, which gives the baby more space and therefore a better position in the belly.

Connecting to one's breath during practice stimulates the parasympathetic nervous system, which increases the production of "feel good" hormones, reduces the production of stress hormones, and improves the reproductive system's functioning—including pregnancy and labor.

Yoga encourages the mind to be present and in the moment, which has been shown to be effective in increasing pain tolerance.

Q. Should pregnant expatriate women be aware of any particular considerations or modifications when practicing yoga in a new country?

A. I believe that when women move countries, they might feel shy about expressing how they feel because they're getting used to a new culture and practices. But if something during the yoga practice doesn't feel good or right in their bodies, it's important for them to be comfortable communicating that to the teacher and stepping back to take rest. It doesn't matter where they are in the world; they should do only what feels good to them and speak up otherwise. They shouldn't feel shy, ashamed, or intimidated by the new culture.

Q. What advice do you have for beginners who have never practiced yoga before but are interested in starting during their pregnancy?

A. If you have never practiced yoga before and would like to start during pregnancy, search for an experienced prenatal yoga teacher. I believe that's the most important thing. They'll be able to tell you what to expect from the class and guide you safely through the practice. Make sure you're cleared by your midwife or doctor before starting any new physical activity during pregnancy.

Q. How can prenatal yoga contribute to building a sense of community and support among expectant mothers in a foreign country?

A. A prenatal yoga class is completely different from any other class. Besides wanting to practice yoga, everyone in the room has something else in common. They're all in a special stage of life: pregnancy. This fact invites all sorts of topics around pregnancy and delivery to class, and these can be pretty intimate subjects, which creates a deeper connection among the students.

MARINA FERRARI | DIETITIAN AND LACTATION CONSULTANT IBCLC[1]

Q. What are the main difficulties new mothers face when starting breastfeeding, and how can they overcome them?

A. The most common challenges at the start of breastfeeding are related to unrealistic expectations about how lactation works and how babies behave, especially during the early weeks. Difficulties with positioning for a comfortable and efficient feed are also common.

Ideally, gathering reliable information before the baby arrives is the best way to prepare, and it goes far beyond knowing the benefits of breastfeeding. It's important to understand what to expect during the first few weeks, know how to identify early signs that something is off, and figure out where to seek help to make necessary adjustments. These considerations become especially important in countries where breastfeeding rates are low, suggesting that breastfeeding support in that context is limited and finding effective help may be more challenging.

Q. Can you share some tips to ensure the baby is latching correctly and feeding efficiently?

A. Especially with newborns, some signs of a good latch are:

- The baby's chin is "indenting" the breast.

- Both of the baby's cheeks look full and are touching the breast.

- The lower lip (if visible) is turned outward.

---

1   IBCLC – International Board-Certified Lactation Consultant

- The areola (if visible) is showing more above the baby's upper lip than below the lower lip (which is likely hidden by the chin).

- The nipple does not appear flattened immediately after feeding.

Signs of effective feedings include:

- The baby doesn't fall asleep shortly after the start of feeding.

- The baby wakes up and wants to feed as often as 10 to 12 times every 24 hours, day and night, during the first month.

- The baby urinates and defecates as frequently as expected for their age.

- The baby regains his or her birth weight within the first two weeks of life and gains weight adequately thereafter.

- Feeds are painless for the mother.

It's important to mention that a baby wanting to nurse approximately every one to two hours during the first month of life or having periods of cluster feedings are normal and expected behaviors.

Q. What do you recommend for mothers who need to return to work but want to continue breastfeeding?

A. The breastfeeding plan upon returning to work will depend on the mother's wishes, the baby's age, whether the baby is already consuming solid foods for nutrition, the commute time and work schedule, the opportunities provided by the mother's workplace, and the local breastfeeding protection legislation. It is suggested that mothers of babies who are exclusively or predominantly breastfed start the plan of pumping and storage one to two weeks before returning to work. If a breast pump will be used, its efficiency should be tested early. This phase is temporary and lasts until the baby's nutrition and hydration through solids and water are sufficient to maintain the baby's well-being during the mother's work shift. It's important to consider the mother's wishes regarding the continuation of breastfeeding.

Q. How can mothers take care of their own health and well-being while breastfeeding?

A. Ideally, maternal health and well-being will primarily come from the care they receive from their support network, rather than from their own actions. However, for immigrant or expatriate mothers, the support network takes different forms. Instead of relying on in-person help from family and friends, support through things like cleaning services, babysitters, and food and grocery delivery can be part of it. The puerperium is a time to accept being cared for! Asking for and willingly receiving help might be the best approach for self-care. Having support for daily practical tasks can automatically create space for moments of well-being and recovery, like taking a shower with enough time to wash your hair, going for a walk, or eating while the food is still hot. These are simple activities which have a very different value once you have children.

I usually encourage families, particularly immigrants or expatriates with limited support networks, to prepare for the postpartum period during pregnancy. This preparation may include stocking the freezer with nutritious meals and familiarizing themselves with available services like those mentioned above. During breastfeeding, gradually resuming social connections, engaging in enjoyable physical activity, consuming nourishing meals, and attending health checks are relevant for overall health, as at any other stage of life.

Q. Should mothers avoid or adopt any certain foods or practices to ensure healthy milk production?

A. Responsive feeding is the best approach for good milk supply. Under normal health conditions, milk supply tends to regulate with the frequency and the amount of breast milk removal. Anything that actively limits the frequency or duration of milk removal can negatively impact the supply, such as pacifier use, setting a feeding schedule, and practices to extend the baby's sleep time. Milk supply is not influenced by the mother's diet—evidence does not suggest that specific foods or drinks can influence it. Sleeping many hours in a row is not required for a good milk supply either, but it's important that mothers allow themselves several periods of rest around the clock, with or without naps. Again, the importance of a support network and adjusting expectations about how much can be done in a day when caring for a baby is emphasized, regardless of the feeding method.

DR. BIANCA NOSÉ, OBSTETRICIAN | GYNECOLOGIST

Q. **What are the signs and symptoms of pregnancy complications that expectant mothers should watch for, especially when they are in a foreign healthcare system?**

A. When you're pregnant and operating under a foreign healthcare system, it's really important to be tuned into your body and aware of any changes that might signal trouble. Here are some symptoms that you should keep an eye on:

1. Vaginal Bleeding: Even a little bleeding can be a warning sign. It's worth getting checked out right away.

2. Severe Nausea and Vomiting: Morning sickness is common, but if it gets severe, it can be a sign of something more serious like hyperemesis gravidarum, which needs medical attention.

3. High Fever: High fever can be a sign of an infection, which isn't just a concern for you but can also affect your baby.

4. Changes in Vaginal Discharge: If your discharge changes in color or consistency or starts to smell bad, it might indicate an infection or that labor is starting too early.

5. Persistent Abdominal Pain: Any constant or very painful sensations in your stomach should be taken seriously—it could be a sign of something like the placenta detaching too early.

6. Swelling: Swelling in your face, hands, or feet could indicate preeclampsia, a serious condition that raises your blood pressure and can affect both you and your baby.

7. Headaches: Bad headaches that don't go away, especially if you're also seeing spots or your vision is blurry, can be a symptom of high blood pressure during pregnancy.

8. Decrease in Baby Movements: If you feel like your baby is moving less than usual, it's a good idea to talk to a doctor. It could be a sign that your baby is in distress.

9. Water Breaking Prematurely: If you think your water has broken early, it's time to head to the hospital.

10. Dizziness or Fainting: Feeling unusually dizzy or fainting could be a result of low blood pressure or something else that needs checking out.

Being in a different country means you need to be proactive about your health care. Keep emergency numbers on hand and know where the nearest hospital with maternity services is located. Always keep your medical records easily accessible and communicate openly with your healthcare providers. Don't hesitate to ask questions or express concerns, even for things that might seem small.

Note: In many countries, dialing either 112 (used in Europe and parts of Asia) or 911 (used mostly in the Americas) can connect you to emergency services.[27]

Q. How can expectant mothers ensure good communication and understanding with their healthcare professionals when language and cultural barriers are a problem?

A. In a new country, we often face the fear of communication, especially with healthcare professionals. To ensure effective communication with healthcare providers in another country, consider learning the local language, or at least basic health-related phrases and terms related to your pregnancy.

If learning the language isn't possible, use interpretation services, whether online or provided by the hospital or health clinic. Many hospitals offer translation services for non-native speakers.

Another important tip is to always have someone accompany you. If this person speaks the local language, that's even better. If not, they can still help you understand instructions and ask questions.

Before medical appointments and exams, write down a list of questions and concerns in a notebook to ensure you don't forget anything. Don't hesitate to clarify if you don't understand something, especially during pregnancy. It's so important to fully understand the guidance and information related to your health and your baby's health. In this case, using a translator app or a person can be very helpful.

Lastly, always try to provide as much information as possible about your medical history and current symptoms, even if they seem irrelevant or unimportant to you. The more information you can provide the better!

DR. PRISCILA ZANOTTI STAGLIORIO | PEDIATRICIAN

Q. What are the most common health concerns for newborns and young children that expatriate parents should be aware of in a new country?

A. Caring for newborns is generally consistent worldwide, with some local variations. In colder regions, respiratory diseases spread more due to enclosed spaces. In hot, humid areas, avoid sun exposure for babies less than six months old during peak hours, and use sunscreen and mosquito repellent for those over six months. For babies with sensitive skin or infants less than six months old, consult a local pediatrician for appropriate products. Hydration is important in humid climates; watch for dehydration signs like reduced urination, sunken eyes, dry lips, low saliva, and tearless crying. For newborns, a sunken fontanelle can indicate dehydration. Ensure babies are not overdressed to prevent overheating and dehydration.

Understand local customs like visiting newborns, holding the baby, or taking babies to events. Avoid plane or car travel that changes atmospheric pressure until the baby is at least a year old.

In some countries, routine follow-ups are rare, and parents rely on emergency care. Others focus on prevention with regular check-ups. Stay informed about disease outbreaks and consult a trusted pediatrician if your child shows signs of illness. If contact with your doctor isn't possible, seek emergency care. Lastly, monitor your child's mental health and be alert to subtle signs.

Q. How can expatriate parents ensure their children receive the necessary vaccinations and healthcare in a foreign country? Might specific vaccines be required or recommended based on the region?

A. Before moving to or vacationing in a new country, research the local healthcare system. In many places, healthcare is private or insurance-based, with limited public services. Ensure you have access to reliable healthcare, including pediatricians, hospitals, and emergency services. Find a trusted pediatrician through referrals and verify their credentials on local medical regulation websites.

For children on continuous medication, bring a one-to-two-month supply with a prescription until you find a local pediatrician to continue treatment. Other necessary medications should also be prescribed locally. For example, Brazilian pediatricians are available who can provide consultations online, making it easier to communicate. Always try to have the same pediatrician for continuity of care, but telemedicine with Brazilian pediatricians is also an option for guidance.

Research required vaccines before moving, and update the vaccination record upon arrival. This task may often require translation. Some vaccines may be mandatory for school attendance, and public schools may require an annual medical report. Consult with a pediatrician about vaccines, the presence of common transmissible diseases, and parasitic diseases transmitted by worms and mosquitoes. Check whether vaccines given in your country meet local requirements, as brands, doses, and intervals may vary.

Q. What advice do you have for parents trying to balance their home country's dietary habits with local food practices for their children?

A. Balancing your home country's diet with local foods can be tough. Start by maintaining your traditional diet, sourcing ingredients from stores that carry products from your home country. For example, Brazilian mothers can look for stores that carry Brazilian items. If that's not feasible, gradually introduce local foods, one at a time, in small quantities. Encourage your child to explore these new foods by involving them in the process—from handling the food before cooking to tasting it once it is prepared.

As both a doctor and a mother, I find the most effective approach is to involve your child in meal setup. Arrange all foods at the center of the table, serve small portions on your child's plate, and let everyone eat without pressuring the child to finish their meal. If the child doesn't eat much, try again in a couple of hours when they show signs of hunger, again without pressure.

DANIELE OLIVEIRA RIBEIRO | CLINICAL PSYCHOLOGIST

Q. What are the most common emotional challenges that expatriate mothers face during pregnancy and postpartum?

A. Anxiety, loneliness, and lack of support are common among migrant mothers. Coming from highly relational and collective cultures, where postpartum support involves other women, caregivers, and family members, these mothers feel a significant gap. Gonçalves's studies (2005) on anxiety and social support in immigrant pregnant women concluded that these women experience high anxiety levels and lower satisfaction with social support. Other common challenges include:

- Mourning life changes and career breaks

- Cultural shock and frustration with differing childbirth and maternity care practices

- Acculturation stress due to the loss of familiar parenting styles or the need to fully adapt to a new cultural perspective on pregnancy

- Identity crises due to changes in relationship roles, bodily changes, lifestyle adjustments, and the subjective and individual relationship with motherhood

- Hormonal changes and their impact on mood

- Mental overload and accumulating responsibilities due to the lack of a support network abroad

Q. How can expectant mothers deal with anxiety and stress during pregnancy in a foreign country?

A. The context of migration needs to be considered, as it acts as a stress factor among expectant mothers. Seek an assessment that takes into account the entire context—your life before migration, current conditions, and available emotional, physical, social, and spiritual resources. Anxiety always arises when we feel in danger, vulnerable, or incapable of experiencing certain life events.

We could say that the first step is to seek a competent professional network to support a pregnant migrant. Research the services offered in your country or local area, which may include: psychologists, therapists, pelvic physiotherapists, lactation consultants, or doulas.

A therapist or psychologist can provide psychological prenatal care facilitating the process of the pregnant woman as she matures to cope with the changes that will occur during pregnancy, labor, and the postpartum period.

When seeking help from a healthcare professional, make sure they have what we call cultural sensitivity, meaning they shouldn't have an ethnocentric and prejudiced view. Receiving support from culturally sensitive healthcare professionals means that the pregnant migrant's culture is respected. This consideration helps prevent misdiagnoses and makes her feel more secure in practicing maternal care according to both her culture of origin and that of the host country. It's important to consult professionals who are open to negotiation and communication. Often, it may be necessary to involve a translator and/or cultural mediator to facilitate communication between the healthcare professional and the pregnant woman.

Another recommendation is to build a social support network and maintain contact with people who promote trust and security. You can do this by looking for mother groups that engage in various activities like physical exercise, picnics, playdates, etc. You can find these groups on social networks like Facebook, Instagram, or apps like Peanuts App.

In cases where anxiety is diagnosed, we recommend that the pregnant woman undergo therapeutic follow-up, establish a healthy routine with the help of her husband or companion, and create a plan for lifestyle changes and for the arrival of the new family member. The more structured the nest is, the more secure the pregnant woman will feel, thus helping to ease her anxiety.

Suggestions that can also help with anxiety and stress management include:

- Investing in an integrative self-care plan (mind/body/social/spiritual/cultural)

- Therapy

- Meditation and mindfulness

- Adapted physical activities for pregnant women

- Cultural, social, and/or spiritual connection activities

- Rest

Q. What strategies can I use to build an emotional support network in a new country?

A. Given that we come from a highly relational and collective culture, mothers who stay in contact with other mothers and social spaces tend to be happier. In these spaces, new friendships form, and mothers can learn new care practices and information to ease their day-to-day life in a new country.

Without the family support network from home, they must create a new circle of connections through group participation, school activities, and in-person events in this new phase of life. Consider post-birth planning with your partner, including household responsibilities, baby care organization, and identifying additional resources for assistance.

Some migrant mothers bring in family members from their home country to help, while others share duties with their partners or hire external support. Joining support groups and seeking online psychology professionals specializing in motherhood and immigration can also be helpful, though in-person participation remains necessary. If you're living in isolated places with few in-person spaces, consider creating your own groups. Organize local community meetups, craft activities, cultural celebrations, picnics, playdates, and activities promoting cultural identity and language preservation for various cultures.

Q. How can cultural change affect mental health during pregnancy and motherhood?

A. During pregnancy, the fetus and mother are influenced by local cultural practices. Each culture has its own unique codes, values, and perspectives on childbirth, as well as varying attitudes toward the role of pain in the birthing process. Cultural perspectives influence breastfeeding, maternity leave duration, and whether the mother works outside the home. Cultural differences in parenting styles impact migrant mothers, leading to acculturation—a cultural perspective change through new cultural contact. This change can either integrate and foster growth or lead to "de-acculturation," where the mother feels deeply uprooted, insecure, and anxious. Disconnection occurs when the mother doesn't identify with her original or new cultural references, leading to isolation and potential mental health issues like depression, anxiety, or panic attacks.

Q. What warning signs of postpartum depression should I look out for, and when should I seek professional help?

A. Even before childbirth, expectant mothers and their partners need to receive support to prepare for the arrival of their new family member. Psychological prenatal care, alongside physical prenatal care, is highly recommended. When a mother receives such support during pregnancy and it continues into postpartum, it can prevent postpartum depression and other mental health issues. Laura Gutman describes postpartum as a time when a mother faces her deepest fears and pains. Every woman needs to be supported during postpartum.

Differentiate baby blues from postpartum depression. Baby blues, which affects 80% to 90% of mothers, is a normal reaction during the first week postpartum and usually resolves on its own. Postpartum depression, starting from the fourth to eighth week postpartum (sometimes later within the first year), can last over a year. Symptoms include irritability, frequent crying, feelings of helplessness, lack of energy, disinterest in sex, changes in eating and sleeping patterns, and physical complaints without apparent organic cause. Symptoms may also include headaches, back pain, vaginal issues, and abdominal pain (Klaus et al., 2000). Postpartum depression symptoms resemble non-pregnancy-related depressive episodes, including mood instability and excessive concern for the baby's well-being.

If you feel the need for support during postpartum, even without severe depression symptoms, seek psychological help. If the mother resists seeking support, or if any new symptoms appear, intervention to guide her toward professional help and building a support network is often necessary.

MARIANE ZAMBONI | NUTRITIONIST

Q. What are the main nutritional needs for pregnant women, and how can women ensure they're meeting those needs, especially when living abroad?

A. All women should receive quality healthcare and nutrition during pregnancy to support the baby's growth and development.

Nutritional requirements rise during this period to sustain both the baby's and the mother's metabolism. Recommendations should be tailored to each woman's lifestyle. For pregnant women living abroad, nutritional guidelines should follow the same principles to reduce risks of complications and ensure the baby's health.

A balanced diet should include adequate calories, proteins, carbohydrates, vitamins, and minerals. Nutritional needs can be met by consuming high-biological-value proteins from animal sources (meat, chicken, eggs, fish), dairy products (milk, cheese, yogurt), and plant-based proteins (beans, lentils, chickpeas, peas). It's important to supplement food with folic acid and iron and to consume foods rich in these nutrients, such as whole grains, dark green vegetables, and legumes.

Hydration is imperative, including water and foods rich in liquids like soups, salads, and fruits. Salt intake should be limited; use herbs like oregano, parsley, chives, thyme, cilantro, and basil instead. In countries like the USA, be mindful of processed foods with high sodium content. Avoid alcohol to prevent fetal alcohol syndrome, which can lead to developmental issues. Nutritional needs also include managing weight gain and preventing gestational hypertension and diabetes. A nutritionist can provide comprehensive support alongside prenatal care.

Q. **How can expatriate mothers manage different food cultures to maintain a balanced and healthy diet during pregnancy?**

A. Expatriate mothers can follow their traditional dietary habits, adjusted to meet pregnancy nutritional needs. Focus on variety by including colorful vegetables, at least three or four servings of fruit daily, lean proteins, eggs, dairy, and moderate carbohydrates, while reducing sugar intake. Fresh, local, and seasonal foods are ideal. Weekly shopping for fresh produce, particularly dark green and orange-yellow vegetables, can ensure a rich intake of iron, folic acid, and vitamin A. In industrialized countries, avoid processed and ultra-processed foods. Preparing meals at home from fresh ingredients is the best choice for both mother and baby.

Q. **What are some common dietary myths or misconceptions that pregnant women should be aware of and avoid?**

A. When a woman finds out she's pregnant, many doubts and myths can arise. Can you eat eggs? Yes, eggs are very nutritious, but always consume them cooked, to avoid contamination. Avoid raw foods like carpaccio, raw kibbeh, and sashimi due to contamination risks. The myth that a pregnant woman should eat for two is widespread, but excessive weight gain can actually cause complications. The caloric increase during pregnancy is individualized, but generally it should be only about 300 kcal a day. Cornmeal and dark beer do not increase breast milk production; proper rest, nutrition, and hydration do. Food cravings are normal due to hormonal changes, but they don't affect the baby's health. Limit coffee to once a day to avoid complications.

Q. How can a balanced diet influence the health and development of the baby during pregnancy?

A. A healthy pregnancy and baby depend on a balanced diet full of the essential vitamins, minerals, and nutrients necessary for the baby's neurodevelopment and formation. Such a diet also maintains the mother's health and aids in postpartum recovery and breastfeeding. Proper nutrition prevents excessive weight gain, hypertension, and gestational diabetes, whereas maternal nutritional imbalance can increase the risk of the child becoming overweight or developing metabolic syndrome and diabetes in the future.

Q. Do you have any tips to help mothers deal with cravings and food aversions during pregnancy, especially while they're living in a country with different culinary traditions?

A. During pregnancy, sudden cravings and food aversions are common. Try to maintain healthy habits; if cravings are unusual and could harm your health, seek help through meditation, breathing exercises, physical activity, massages, and relaxation techniques, as these cravings can be linked to maternal anxiety and emotions. A balanced diet with appropriate supplementation can help control cravings as well. Have four to five small meals a day, at three-hour intervals. Avoid large quantities at once, chew well, and include fruits, vegetables, proteins, and carbohydrates. When living abroad, opt for foods with less fat, condiments, peppers, and salt. These habits favor the mother's good digestion.

GABRIELA TELES | LAWYER

Q. What are the main legal challenges that expatriate parents face when trying to obtain citizenship or visas for their newborns in a foreign country?

A. Expatriate parents should always check the local laws and regulations related to birth registration, citizenship, and visa requirements. They must understand the specific documentation needed and the processes involved, which can be complex and vary significantly from one country to another. Consulting a local legal expert or an immigration lawyer can provide valuable guidance and ensure that all necessary steps are correctly followed.

Because I work in Portugal, I can provide some specific information about this country. From 2020, babies born in Portugal to parents who legally reside here or who have been residing for more than a year, even without a residence permit, are entitled to Portuguese nationality. This nationality is granted at the time of birth registration at the IRN or at the *Nascer Cidadão* desks located in maternity hospitals across the country. Parents are required to register babies not entitled to Portuguese nationality at these desks as foreigners. Subsequently, the baby's nationality must be registered at the consulate or embassy of the parents' home country, with the required documents.

Q. What documents and evidence do parents need to prepare and present when applying for citizenship or permanent residency for their children in a new country?

A. Immigrant parents must be aware of the destination country's specific requirements when applying for citizenship or permanent residency. Portugal, for example, has many possibilities for regularization for both adults and children. Normally, children can be reunited with parents who already hold a visa or residence permit. However, in some cases, a child may obtain a residence permit independently, such as when he or she is studying in the country. In this scenario, the parents may later qualify for a residence permit based on their responsibility for the child's education and support. While each type of visa has its own requirements, one document is always necessary for minors: the updated, authenticated, and translated birth certificate. I always recommend planning and consulting with a qualified professional to ensure the family's regularization process goes smoothly.

Q. Are expatriate children entitled to specific benefits or legal protections when moving to a new country?

A. Parents should be informed about the rights and benefits available to ensure their children receive all the necessary support. In Portugal, children have extensive legal protection and access to healthcare and education. Regardless of the parents' legal residency status, pregnant women (who have been in Portugal for more than 90 days) and children can access the Portuguese healthcare system for free, for various services including pregnancy monitoring, childbirth, and child development follow-up. Additionally, families within the fourth income bracket of the IRS (income tax) are entitled to the Child Benefit (*Abono de Família*).

Q. What advice would you give to expatriate parents planning an international move, to ensure a smooth legal transition and minimize the risk of immigration complications?

A. Expatriate parents must prepare adequately for the move by researching and understanding all of the destination country's legal requirements. Consulting an immigration specialist or a local lawyer can be very helpful to ensure that all necessary documents and procedures are properly followed and to minimize the risk of complications. Unfortunately, in Portugal, we observe many cases of arbitrary denial of rights. Often, if a person doesn't know their rights, they accept the denial and miss out on accessing them. It's so important to be well-informed, to seek the help of qualified professionals to enter the country legally, and to know your rights, especially when immigrating or moving with children and babies.

DÁGILA SCOPARO | PELVIC PHYSIOTHERAPIST

Q. What are the main challenges that expatriate women face regarding pelvic health during pregnancy and postpartum?

A. Cultural Differences

- Taboos and Stigmas: In some cultures, issues related to pelvic and sexual health can be considered taboo, making it difficult to seek treatment and support due to shame or lack of sexual education.

- Traditional Practices and Beliefs: Certain cultural practices or beliefs can influence women's perceptions of the need for specific pelvic health care, both in their own country and abroad.

Access to Healthcare

- Unfamiliar Healthcare System: Understanding a new healthcare system can be confusing and intimidating. Women may not be aware of the available services or how to access them.

- Health Insurance Coverage: Issues related to health insurance, such as limited coverage or lack of knowledge about how to obtain insurance, can hinder access to necessary care.

Language Barriers

- Communication with Healthcare Professionals: Language difficulties can impede effective communication with healthcare professionals, leading to inaccurate diagnoses or limited understanding of treatment instructions.

- Education and Information: The lack of educational materials in the patient's native language can limit access to important information about pelvic health and necessary care.

Social Isolation

- Lack of Family and Community Support: The absence of a supportive family and community network can increase stress and feelings of isolation, negatively affecting mental and physical health.

- Difficulty Forming New Support Networks: Adapting to a new country can be lonely, making it hard to form new connections that can provide emotional and practical support.

Differences in Standard Care

- Variations in Treatment Protocols: Treatment protocols and standard practices can vary significantly between countries, causing confusion or distrust about the treatments offered.

- Different Expectations: Expectations regarding care during pregnancy and postpartum can differ, leading to potential dissatisfaction or frustration with the care received.

Mental and Emotional Health

- Stress and Anxiety: Moving to a new country, especially during pregnancy or the postpartum period, can increase stress and anxiety levels, which can impact overall and pelvic health.

- Postpartum Depression: The risk of postpartum depression can be exacerbated by isolation, lack of support, and cultural adaptation challenges.

Q. What practices or exercises would you recommend for strengthening the pelvic floor during pregnancy, especially for those who may not have easy access to pelvic therapy in their new country?

A. To be effective and deliver results, whether in person or online, Pelvic Floor Muscle Training (PFMT) requires a preliminary evaluation. Exercise protocols are individualized based on each patient's needs, so generalized exercises may not only fail to resolve your issue but could also worsen your condition.

For example, an evaluation can determine whether your muscles are weak, lack endurance, lack coordination, are tense, or any combination of these conditions. Individualized treatment will be based on each patient's specific response.

Additional Tips:

- Consistency: Regular practice of exercises is essential for improvement.

- Breathing: Breathe naturally; don't hold your breath, and don't keep your abdomen contracted all the time!

- Mobility: Keep your pelvis moving with simple exercises or even some fun dancing!

- In the Bathroom: When using the bathroom, relax during bowel movements and urination.

- Pelvic Exercises: Do pelvic muscle exercises regularly.

- Stay Hydrated: Keep yourself well-hydrated to promote overall health and tissue elasticity.

- Mind Your Posture: Pay attention to your posture throughout the day, as good posture helps reduce pressure on the pelvic floor.

- Balanced Diet: Maintain a balanced diet and make healthy choices to ensure the proper functioning of your bladder and bowel.

- Avoid High-Impact Exercises: Steer clear of high-impact exercises that might overload the pelvic floor.

These simple and accessible tips can help keep your body active and support the proper functioning of the pelvic floor during pregnancy.

Q. What are signs that a woman should seek the help of a pelvic physiotherapist during pregnancy or postpartum? How can a professional evaluation help prevent future problems?

A. Signs that a woman should seek the help of a pelvic physiotherapist are:

Urinary or Fecal Incontinence

- Involuntary loss of urine when coughing, sneezing, laughing, or during physical activities

- Difficulty controlling bowel movements

Pelvic or Lower Back Pain

- Persistent pain in the pelvic region, lower back, upper back, or buttocks

- Discomfort when walking, sitting, or performing daily activities

Pelvic Organ Prolapse

- Feeling of heaviness or pressure in the pelvis

- Sensation of something "falling" or a "ball" coming out of the vagina

Sexual Dysfunction

- Pain during sexual intercourse (dyspareunia)

- Feeling of looseness or decreased sexual pleasure

Difficulty in Activating or Relaxing Pelvic Floor Muscles

- Feeling of weakness or inability to contract the pelvic floor muscles

- Difficulty in completely relaxing the pelvic floor muscles

Painful or Sensitive Scars

- Painful or sensitive scars from an episiotomy or cesarean section

- Formation of adhesions or scar tissue that causes discomfort

Changes in Posture and Mobility

- Postural changes due to pregnancy that cause discomfort or pain

- Limitation of movement or difficulty performing daily activities

How a professional evaluation can help prevent future problems:

- Accurate Diagnosis: A detailed evaluation by a pelvic physiotherapist can identify specific problems and provide an accurate diagnosis.

- Personalized Treatment Plan: Based on the evaluation, the physiotherapist can create a personalized treatment plan to meet the individual patient's needs.

- Education and Body Awareness: The patient learns about the anatomy and function of the pelvic floor, along with strategies to prevent future problems.

- Prevention of Complications: Early intervention can prevent serious complications such as severe prolapse or chronic incontinence.

Treatment and Rehabilitation

- Manual techniques to relieve pain, improve tissue mobility, and promote healing

- Instruction in strengthening and relaxation exercises for the pelvic floor muscles

- Biofeedback and Electrotherapy: Use of technologies to assist in muscle re-education and improve pelvic floor function

- Posture and Ergonomics Guidance: Advice on maintaining good posture and performing daily activities without overloading the pelvic floor

- Training in behavior modification techniques to support pelvic floor health

REFERENCES

1. Evans, A. (2022). The 4 Types of Healthcare System Designs and Structures. [online] GoodRx. Available at: https://www.goodrx.com/hcp-articles/providers/healthcare-system-designs [Accessed 8 Jul. 2024].

2. Vankar, P. (2023). Trust in healthcare by country 2022. [online] Statista. Available at: https://www.statista.com/statistics/1071027/trust-levels-towards-healthcare-in-select-countries/ [Accessed 8 Jul. 2024].

3. Japan Health Policy NOW (n.d.). Japan Health Policy NOW – Health Insurance System. [online] Japan Health Policy NOW. Available at: https://japanhpn.org/en/hs1/.

4. Dept. of Health and Human Services Office on Women's Health (2019). Prenatal Care. [online] Medlineplus.gov. Available at: https://medlineplus.gov/prenatalcare.html [Accessed 27 Jun. 2024].

5. www.hematology.org. (n.d.). Anemia and Pregnancy. [online] Available at: https://www.hematology.org/education/patients/anemia/pregnancy#:~:text=Many%20of%20the%20symptoms%20of [Accessed 12 Jul. 2024].

6. William Russell. (n.d.). How Much Does Average Expat Health Insurance Cost? [online] Available at: https://www.william-russell.com/international-health-insurance/how-much-does-expat-health-insurance-cost/.

7. GOV.UK. (n.d.). Parental rights and responsibilities. [online] Available at: https://www.gov.uk/parental-rights-responsibilities/who-has-parental-responsibility#:~:text=A%20mother%20automatically%20has%20parental [Accessed 27 Jun. 2024].

8. Make it in Germany (n.d.). Financial support for families. [online] www.make-it-in-germany.com. Available at: https://www.make-it-in-germany.com/en/living-in-germany/family-life/financial-support-families#:~:text=During%20parental%20leave%2C%20you%20will [Accessed 6 Jun. 2024].

9. Vucendic, U. (2022). Countries With the Best Maternity and Paternity Leave. [online] Vacation Tracker. Available at: https://vacationtracker.io/blog/countries-with-the-best-maternity-and-paternity-leave/ [Accessed 17 Jul. 2024].

10. Backes, E.P. and Scrimshaw, S.C. (2020). Maternal and Newborn Care in the United States. [online] www.ncbi.nlm.nih.gov. National Academies Press (US). Available at: https://www.ncbi.nlm.nih.gov/books/NBK555484/ [Accessed 1 Jun. 2024]

11. McCool, W.F. and Simeone, S.A. (2002). Birth in the United States: an overview of trends past and present. Nursing Clinics of North America, [online] 37(4), pp.735–746. doi:https://doi.org/10.1016/s0029-6465(02)00020-8.

12. Filipovic, J. (2014). Inside the war on natural birth, where c-sections are a status symbol and 'choice' is a myth | Jill Filipovic. The Guardian. [online] 10 Apr. Available at: https://www.theguardian.com/commentisfree/2014/apr/10/natural-birth-c-section-choice-brazil-forced-pregnancy [Accessed 1 Jun. 2024].

13. Solanki, G.C., Cornell, J.E., Daviaud, E. and Fawcus, S. (2020). Caesarean section rates in South Africa: A case study of the health systems challenges for the proposed National Health Insurance. South African Medical Journal, 110(8), p.747. doi:https://doi.org/10.7196/samj.2020.v110i8.14699.

14. anderker, A. (2021). C-section rate among South African medical scheme members the highest in the world. [online] Daily Maverick. Available at: https://www.dailymaverick.co.za/opinionista/2021-09-05-c-section-rate-among-south-african-medical-scheme-members-the-highest-in-the-world/#:~:text=Across%20the%20world%2C%20however%2C%20researchers [Accessed 1 Jun. 2024].

15. Focus, E. (2023). Italy - Maternity and Giving Birth. [online] Expat Focus. Available at: https://www.expatfocus.com/italy/guide/italy-maternity-and-giving-birth [Accessed 27 Jun. 2024].

16. AABC American Association of Birth Centers (n.d.). Birth Centers are Growing - American Association Of Birth Centers. [online] www.birthcenters.org. Available at: https://www.birthcenters.org/birth-centers-are-growing [Accessed 30 May 2024].

17. Bondolfi, S. (2018). The rift between natural birth and on-demand C-sections. [online] SWI swissinfo.ch. Available at: https://www.swissinfo.ch/eng/society/how-the-swiss-give-birth_the-rift-between-natural-birth-and-on-demand-c-sections/44308680#:~:text=Birth%20centres%3A%20Giving%20birth%20in [Accessed 30 May 2024].

18. van den Berg, S. (2024). Home birth in the Netherlands: why the Dutch cherish them. [online] Expatica. Available at: https://www.expatica.com/nl/healthcare/womens-health/home-births-in-the-netherlands-100749/#dutch-women [Accessed 1 Jun. 2024].

19. www.medicalnewstoday.com. (2018). Foley bulb induction: What it is and what to expect. [online] Available at: https://www.medicalnewstoday.com/articles/322956#:~:text=When%20the%20balloon%20inflates%20inside [Accessed 25 Jul. 2024].

20. Teen, L. (2021). The Very Best Relaxation and Breathing Techniques for Labor. [online] Mommy Labor Nurse. Available at: https://mommylabornurse.com/breathing-techniques-labor/ [Accessed 12 Jul. 2024].

21. Mayo Clinic Staff (2023). Labor positions. [online] Mayo Clinic. Available at: https://www.mayoclinic.org/healthy-lifestyle/labor-and-delivery/in-depth/labor/art-20546804 [Accessed 17 Jul. 2024].

22. American Pregnancy Association. (2017). Water Births. [online] Available at: https://americanpregnancy.org/healthy-pregnancy/labor-and-birth/water-births/#:~:text=Benefits%20for%20Mother%3A&text=Buoyancy%20promotes%20more%20efficient%20uterine [Accessed 17 Jul. 2024].

23. Mayo Clinic. (2023). Video: The epidural block. [online] Available at: https://www.mayoclinic.org/healthy-lifestyle/labor-and-delivery/multimedia/vbac/vid-20084704 [Accessed 17 Jul. 2024].

24. American Pregnancy Association. (2012). Spinal Block. [online] Available at: https://americanpregnancy.org/healthy-pregnancy/labor-and-birth/spinal-block/ [Accessed 17 Jul. 2024].

25. Admin, A.P.A. (2014). Nitrous Oxide During Labor. [online] American Pregnancy Association. Available at: https://americanpregnancy.org/healthy-pregnancy/labor-and-birth/nitrous-oxide-labor/#:~:text=As%20your%20due%20date%20approaches [Accessed 17 Jul. 2024].

26. nigel.ayres77058500 (2023). Top 6 Strategies To Balance Motherhood While Living Abroad As AnExpat. [online] Expat Network. Available at: https://expatnetwork.com/top-6-strategies-to-balance-motherhood-while-living-abroad-as-an-expat/ [Accessed 8 Jun. 2024].

27. Wikipedia (2024). List of emergency telephone numbers. [online] Wikipedia. Available at: https://en.wikipedia.org/wiki/List_of_emergency_ telephone_numbers#cite_note-lonelyplanet.com-2 [Accessed 2 Jun. 2024].

28. AMERICAN PSYCHIATRIC ASSOCIATION. (2000). Diagnostic and statistical manual of mental disorders (4th ed., text rev.). Washington, D.C.: American Psychiatric Association.

29. COOPER, P. J., & MURRAY, L. (1995). Postnatal depression and child development. The Guilford Press.

30. GONÇALVES, S. (2005). Ansiedade e suporte social em grávidas imigrantes. Monografia, Lisboa, Instituto Superior de Psicologia Aplicada.

31. GUTMAN, Laura. A maternidade e o encontro com a própria sombra [recurso eletrônico]. Tradução Luís Carlos Cabral, Mariana Laura Corullón. 1. ed. Rio de Janeiro: Best Seller, 2016.

32. KLAUS, M. H., KENNELL, J. H., & KLAUS, P. H. (2000). The doula book: How a trained labor companion can help you have a shorter, easier, and healthier birth. Perseus Publishing.

33. SCHMIDT, E. B., PICCOLOTO, N. M., & MÜLLER, M. C. (2005). Depressão pós-parto: fatores de risco e repercussões no desenvolvimento infantil. Psico-USF, 10(1), 61-68.

34. SOPA, M. (2009). Representações e práticas da maternidade em contexto multicultural e migratório. 336 f. Dissertação (Mestrado em Comunicação em Saúde) – Universidade Aberta, Lisboa.

35. RAMOS, Natália (1993) Maternage en milieu portugais autochtone et immigre de la tradition á la modernité. Une étude ethnopsychologique. Tese de Doutoramento em Psicologia, Paris, Universidade René Descartes.

9 782970 184805